# Nuclear Localization of Growth Factors and of Monoclonal Antibodies

**Editor**

**Ewa M. Rakowicz-Szulczynska, Ph.D.**
*University of Nebraska Medical Center*
*Omaha, Nebraska*

CRC Press
Boca Raton   Ann Arbor   London   Tokyo

**Library of Congress Cataloging-in-Publication Data**

Nuclear localization of growth factors and of monoclonal antibodies/
editor Ewa M. Rakowicz-Szulczynska.
  p. cm.
  Includes bibliographical references and index.
  ISBN 0-8493-4713-0
  1. Growth factors — Analysis. 2. Growth factors — Receptors.
3. Monoclonal antibodies. 4. Antinuclear factors. I. Rakowicz
-Szulczynska, Ewa M.
QP552.G76N83 1993
616.99′4079 — dc20                                              93-12471
                                                                  CIP

# PREFACE

Cloning, sequencing, point mutations, transfections, and gene transfer are approaches which mark the trends in modern biology. State of the art techniques and computerized equipment promote rapid progress in understanding the structure and function of protein and nucleic acid molecules. Surprisingly, the general knowledge of cancer cell biology has remained unchanged for years. Earlier studies have followed the well-established, dogmatic view of cell structure and function. The cell interacts with the environment through the mediation of highly specialized cell surface receptors. Each molecule of the exogenous protein hormone, or growth factor, is dogmatically believed to be destined for intracellular degradation, while the wise second messengers, at the command of the tyrosine kinase, transfer the signals from the activated cell surface receptors to the nucleus.

How many laboratories truly have followed the degradation rate of protein molecules internalized by cells? For the last 15 years, my students and collaborators failed to detect total degradation of internalized proteins, since in most cases 3 to 70% of internalized growth factors and 10 to 30% of monoclonal antibodies are detected in a nondegraded form inside the nucleus, in a complex with chromatin. Currently, almost each known growth factor has been reported by at least one laboratory to be localized inside the cell nucleus. For some researchers, nuclear targets for nerve growth factor, fibroblast growth factor, epidermal growth factor, platelet-derived growth factor, or angiotensin represent models for studies on gene regulation. These studies, which do not fit accepted views of cell function, have remained for years on the margin of the mainstream of growth factor research. Our latest discovery that some anti-cancer or anti-HIV antibodies mimic intracellular pathways of growth factors and in a nondegraded form accumulate in the chromatin of target cells convinced me that research leading to understanding the nuclear pathway of exogenous proteins deserves to enter the science through the main door.

Monoclonal antibodies that attach to the chromatin of tumor cells may either directly exert a biological function similar to growth factor molecules or, after conjugation with radioactive ligands, may effectively damage DNA. Future studies may be extended on monoclonal antibody–anti-transcriptional drug conjugates.

I have prepared this book to focus the attention of my research colleagues on some of the neglected steps of cell function which potentially may be crucial for understanding the mechanisms of malignant transformation. When the existing belief in intracytoplasmic degradation of growth factors and other molecules such as monoclonal antibodies is replaced by rational analysis of intracellular pathways of these molecules, then we will have a chance to develop a new generation of drugs targeted to the nucleus of cancer or virus-infected cells.

Usually, a book summarizes well-established research. In our case, this book summarizes some unconventional and highly preliminary data which indicate that the nucleus expresses some unique receptors for growth factors, as well as for monoclonal antibodies directed against cell surface antigens.

*Ewa M. Rakowicz-Szulczynska*

# THE EDITOR

Ewa M. Rakowicz-Szulczynska, Ph.D., D.M.Sc., is Associate Professor and Head of the Laboratory of Molecular Oncology at the Department of Obstetrics and Gynecology, College of Medicine, of the University of Nebraska Medical Center in Omaha, Nebraska. She is also Courtesy Associate Professor of Oncology at the Eppley Institute for Research on Cancer and Allied Diseases, and a Graduate Faculty Member and Graduate College Faculty Fellow of the University of Nebraska.

Dr. Rakowicz-Szulczynska received her M.S. degree from the A. Mickiewicz University in Poznan, Poland, in 1974. She obtained her Ph.D. in biochemistry in 1977, and in 1982 she received the degree of Doctor Habilitate of Medical Sciences in Genetics from the Academy of Medicine, Poznan, Poland. From 1977 to 1984, Dr. Rakowicz-Szulczynska was an Assistant Professor and later Associate Professor at the Institute of Human Genetics of the Polish Academy of Sciences. From 1981 to 1985 she was also the Vice-Director for Scientific Affairs of that institute.

In 1984, Dr. Rakowicz-Szulczynska was appointed by the Wistar Institute of Anatomy and Biology in Philadelphia, Pennsylvania, where she took a new approach to studies on cancer biology, using chromatin antigens as the target. In 1992, she assumed her present position at the University of Nebraska.

Dr. Ewa Rakowicz-Szulczynska is the author of 50 research papers. She has invented two U.S. patents concerning new methods of developing drugs for cancer therapy. She has been invited to present over 60 lectures in Europe and the United States. Her current major research interests concentrate on the etiology and biology of gynecological cancer and on improving diagnostic and therapeutic methods by using unconventional techniques of drug delivery to the cancer cell nucleus.

# CONTRIBUTORS

**F. Amalric, D.Sc.**
Professor
Laboratoire de Biologie
Moleculaire des Eucaryotes
CNRS
Toulouse, France

**V. Baldin, Ph.D.**
Laboratoire de Biologie
Moleculaire des Eucaryotes
CNRS
Toulouse, France

**Gerard Bouche, D.Sc.**
Professor
Laboratoire de Biologie
Moleculaire des Eucaryotes
CNRS
Toulouse, France

**P. Brethenou, Ph.D.**
Laboratoire de Biologie
Moleculaire des Eucaryotes
CNRS
Toulouse, France

**Yves Courtois, D.Sc.**
Unité de Gerontologic
Institute National de la Santé et de la
  Recherche Medicale (INSERM)
Paris, France

**L. Creancier, M.Sc.**
Laboratoire de Biologie
Moleculaire des Eucaryotes
CNRS
Toulouse, France

**Paul J. Durda, Ph.D.**
Immunobiologicals Department
E.I. DuPont de Nemours
North Billerica, Massachusetts
  *formerly*
Senior Scientist
Genzyme Corporation
Cambridge, Massachusetts

**M. Guyader, Ph.D.**
Laboratoire de Biologie
Moleculaire des Eucaryotes
CNRS
Toulouse, France

**Wojciech Kaczmarski, Ph.D.**
The Wistar Institute
Philadelphia, Pennsylvania
  *and*
Institute of Human Genetics
Polish Academy of Sciences
Poznan, Poland

**Ewa M. Rakowicz-Szulczynska, Ph.D.,
D.M.Sc.**
Associate Professor
Department of Obstetrics & Gynecology
University of Nebraska Medical Center
Omaha, Nebraska
  *and*
Courtesy Associate Professor
Eppley Institute for Research on Cancer
  and Allied Diseases
Omaha, Nebraska

**Vic Raso, Ph.D.**
Senior Scientist, Cell and Molecular
  Biology
Boston Biomedical Research Institute
Boston, Massachusetts

**Richard N. Re, M.D.**
Vice President and Director
Division of Research
Alton Ochsner Medical Foundation
New Orleans, Louisiana
  *and*
Head, Section on Hypertensive Diseases
Ochsner Clinic
New Orleans, Louisiana

**A. M. Roman, Ph.D.**
Laboratoire de Biologie
Moleculaire des Eucaryotes
CNRS
Toulouse, France

**Kathelyn S. Steimer, Ph.D.**
Viral Immunobiology Department
Chiron Corporation
Emeryville, California

**Isabelle Truchet, D.Sc.**
Laboratoire de Biologie
Moleculaire des Eucaryotes
CNRS
Toulouse, France

# TABLE OF CONTENTS

*History of Science teaches that*

*studies confirming dogmas*

*find several sponsors,*

*while research denying dogmas*

*brings progress seen in the next generations.*

Ewa M. Rakowicz-Szulczynska

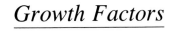

*Growth Factors*

Chapter 1

# CHROMATIN RECEPTORS FOR GROWTH FACTORS

Ewa M. Rakowicz-Szulczynska

## TABLE OF CONTENTS

0-8493-4713-0/94/$0.00 + $.50
© 1994 by CRC Press, Inc.

3

# I. CLASSICAL THEORY OF GROWTH FACTOR ACTION

## A. INTRODUCTION

Growth factors are the low molecular weight proteins that exert pleiotropic effects on a broad range of physiological and pathological processes, such as embryogenesis, cell survival, cell growth and development, hemopoiesis, tissue repair, immune responses, atherosclerosis, and neoplasia.[1-5] Abnormally high expression of the cell surface receptors for growth factors on tumor cells and synthesis of various growth factors by several tumors focused the attention of many laboratories on the role of growth factors in malignant transformation and maintaining the malignant phenotype of cancer cells. The link between growth factors or growth factor receptors and oncogenes strongly suggests that further progress in developing drugs against cancer, as well as against several metabolic diseases, would depend on understanding the mechanism of cell growth regulation by growth factors.

Growth factors recognize specific receptors localized on the cell surface of the target cells. Binding of a growth factor to its receptor results in internalization of the receptor-growth factor complex through the process of receptor-mediated endocytosis. Most researchers believe that after internalization, the cell surface receptor and the growth factor are degraded in the lysosomal system. Alternatively, a possibility of the receptor recycling to the cell surface is considered.[1-3]

The early signals generated in the membrane and in the cytoplasm by the growth factor-activated receptor are propagated into the nucleus, which results in stimulation of DNA synthesis and cell division.[6] Since DNA synthesis represents a late event, occurring 10 to 15 h after cell induction with growth factors, most studies have been concentrated on the early molecular and biochemical events that take place in the cytoplasm after interaction of the growth factor with the receptor.[6-16] The hunt for second messengers which might represent the hypothetical intracellular mediators of growth factor action resulted in a precise biochemical description of several growth factor-activated compounds.

## B. SECOND MESSENGERS

One of the earliest responses to several growth factors is an increase in fluxes of monovalent ions such as $Na^+$, $K^+$, and $H^+$ across the plasma membrane and alkalinization of cytoplasm.[6-8] As early as 15 s after the growth factors' interaction with the target receptor, there is efflux of $Ca^{2+}$ from the cell, which leads to a rapid decrease in the $Ca^{2+}$ content inside the activated cells.[6,9,10,14,15] The mobilization of $Ca^{2+}$ may be mediated by inositol 1,4,5-triphosphate (IP3), which is frequently proposed as a second messenger in growth factor action (reviewed in References 6 and 11). Since IP3 is generated as a product of hydrolysis of phosphatidylinositol 4,5-biphosphate (PIP-2) in the plasma membrane in the process that also generates 1,2-diacylglycerol (DAG), DAG is also proposed as a second messenger. DAG is an activator of proteinase kinase C, which is believed to have a critical role in the action of phorbol esters (tumor promoters).[12,13] Activation of the proteinase kinase C leads to increased activity of $Na^+/H^+$ antiport system.[13] In addition to the biochemical events that follow cell stimulation with different growth factors, some more or less specific effects of particular growth factors are observed. For example, PDGF (but not EGF or insulin) increases the cellular level of cyclic adenosine monophosphate (cAMP).[16,17]

A critical role in cell induction by growth factors is played by tyrosine kinase[1-3,14,15,18] and guanosine 5'-triphosphate (GTP)-binding proteins.[19] Protein kinase activity is exhibited by most of the growth factor receptors. Tyrosine kinase activity of the EGF receptor ($M_r$ 170,000) was one of the earliest discovered.[20-23] Other growth factor receptors, PDGF,[24,25] insulin,[26-28] and insulin-like growth factor I (IGF-I),[29,30] also exhibit tyrosine kinase activity. In the presence of the corresponding growth factor, receptors are autophosphorylated and can catalyze phosphorylation of exogenous substrates *in vitro*. Nerve growth factor receptor was for a long time considered as the receptor which does not express the tyrosine kinase.[31-33] Recent experiments indicated that in addition to a low molecular weight NGF receptor, which does not have the tyrosine kinase domain,[31-33] another high molecular weight receptor represents a product of the tyrosine kinase proto-oncogene.[34-37]

How the signals mediated by the second messengers described above are translocated to the nucleus has not been established. Crouch[38] found that the GTP-binding protein, Gi, in cells stimulated with insulin or EGF, is translocated to the nucleus and binds to the chromatin, which suggests that protein Gi may participate in mediating the signal induced by growth factors to the nucleus. Protein kinase C, which, after induction of NIH/3Tc cells, is translocated to the nuclear envelope and induces phosphorylation of lamins A, B, C, is also considered a mediator of growth factor-induced signal.[39] However, the effect is not only typical for PDGF, but also for phorbol esters.[39] As the nuclear mediators of growth factor action, the products of the cellular oncogenes, c-*myc*, c-*src*, and c-*fos*, are considered.[40-47] However, activation of oncogenes, particularly c-*myc*, is also observed in processes of normal growth and regeneration.[47-50]

## C. REPRESENTATIVE GROWTH FACTORS
## 1. EGF

EGF acts as a mitogen for a variety of cells *in vitro* and *in vivo*.[1-3,51] Its biological activity is mediated by the cell surface receptor ($M_r$ 170,000), which exhibits tyrosine kinase activity.[20-23,51-53] Two affinity classes of EGF receptors were identified,[54,55] the function of which in mediating the cell response to EGF is unknown. After binding of EGF to the cell surface receptor, the receptor-ligand complex is internalized into the cell via the clathrin-coated pits pathway of endocytosis.[56-59] In intact cells, binding of EGF to its receptor activates autocatalytic activity of the tyrosine-kinase towards the EGF receptor.[51-53] Serine and threonine of the receptor also become phosphorylated through the $Ca^{2+}$ and phospholipid-dependent protein kinase C.[60,61] How the mitogenic signal induced by EGF is further transmitted to the nucleus is currently unknown. It was determined that in response to EGF, ribosomal protein S6 and several other cytoplasmic proteins undergo phosphorylation on tyrosine, serine, and threonine.[62-64] It is suggested that phosphorylation of the ribosomal S6 protein may modulate initiation of protein synthesis and thereby affect cell proliferation.[64,65] Analysis of insertional mutants of EGF receptors indicated that tyrosine kinase activity of the EGF receptor is critical for initiation of S6 phosphorylation and induction of DNA synthesis, while it is not required for the process of internalization.[66] Honegger et al.[67] compared the various cell responses, including enhanced expression of c-*fos* and c-*myc*, morphological changes, and stimulation of DNA synthesis, mediated by the wild-type of EGF receptor and of the receptor mutated at Lys-721, which is the critical residue for tyrosine kinase activity. The mutated receptor was unable to activate any of the tested reactions mediated by the wild-type.[62] Although according to the experiments described above,[66,67] tyrosine kinase activity seems to have a critical role in the cell response to EGF, induction of tyrosine kinase activity is not sufficient to stimulate DNA synthesis. Defize et al.[68] found that three monoclonal antibodies (mAbs) against EGF receptor — one against the protein domain and two others against carbohydrate determinants of this receptor — were able to induce tyrosine kinase activity as well as induce receptor clustering, without stimulation of DNA synthesis.

Despite extensive studies on potential second messengers in EGF action, the mechanism of EGF-activated cell division remains unknown. In particular, the biological consequences of EGF receptor and EGF internalization[69] do not yet have a rational explanation.

The EGF receptor shows strong homology with the *erb* B[70-73] and *neu* oncogene products.[74-79] Protooncogene c-*erb* B and the EGF receptor gene are located in a region of human chromosome 7.[71,72] Human protooncogene c-*erb* B1 represents the counterpart of the v-*erb* oncogene of the avian erythroblastosis virus (AEV), which induces erythroblastosis, sarcomas, or carcinomas.[73] Oncogene c-*neu,* which also exhibits homology to the EGF receptor, encodes a 180,000 $M_r$ membrane-bound protein. Oncogene c-*neu* is mainly expressed in breast and ovarian carcinomas.[74,75,77-79] Oncogenes' products, c-*erb* B and c-*neu,* do not bind EGF.[78,80] In addition to EGF, the EGF receptor is recognized and activated by the transforming growth factor α, which is secreted by several tumor cell lines.[81-84] The EGF receptor is overexpressed on several carcinomas: breast,[85-88] bladder,[89] colorectal,[90] vulval,[90-91] and lung;[92] also on melanoma,[93] glioma,[94] sarcoma,[95] and bone tumors.[96] Certain mAb against the EGF receptor block growth of tumors in nude mice.[97,98] mAb 425 against the EGF receptor have already found application in experimental immunotherapy of human gliomas.[99-103]

## 2. PDGF

PDGF is as dimeric glycoprotein ($M_r$ 30,000) which exists in a form of heterodimers consisting of A and B chains, or homodimers A-A or B-B (References 104 to 107; reviewed in Reference 108). Heterodimeric A-B PDGF is produced by human platelets;[104,107,109] porcine PDGF appears to consist of B-B homodimers;[110] and several tumor cell lines produce PDGF A-A homodimers.[110-114] The amino acid sequence of the B chain is identical to that of the part of p28 *sis,* the product of the oncogene v-*sis* of simian sarcoma virus.[115-127] PDGF in all forms is highly mitogenic, and it is suggested that it represents one of the basic growth factors which stimulate autocrine growth of tumors.[128-135] Although different dimeric forms of PDGF are mitogenic, they have different functional activities; PDGF A-A has lower mitogenic activity, chemotactic activity, and ability to cause actin rearrangement than has PDGF-A-B.[136,139] PDGF acts through specific receptors.[140-142] Two types of PDGF receptors exist; the receptor of the A type binds all three forms of PDGF (A-B, A-A, B-B), while the type B receptor binds PDGF B-B with high affinity and PDGF A-B with lower affinity, but does not recognize PDGF A-A.[143,144]

The PDGF receptor of the B type exhibits tyrosine kinase activity, and the molecular weight of this receptor, estimated based on cross-linking with [125]I-PDGF, is approximately 163 to 185 kDa.[143,144] Two forms of PDGF A type receptor were identified: the major component and the minor component, which, according to crosslinking experiments, exhibit 140 and 160 kDa,[143] and, according to gene sequencing and analysis of the product expressed by transfected cos-1 cells, exhibit 160 and 185 kDa, respectively.[144]

Binding of PDGF to the cell surface receptor results in activation of the tyrosine kinase of the receptor,[24,25] and also leads to the production of inositol triphosphate and diacylglycerol.[6,11] Diacylglicerol stimulates protein kinase C, which has been considered the mediator of PDGF action.[145,146] In addition, activation of the PDGF receptor is also associated with induction of protooncogenes c-*myc,* c-*fos,* and c-*src.*[42,43,44,108] Coughlin et al.[147] found, however, that activation of protein kinase C and induction of c-*myc* are not sufficient to exert a mitogenic effect. Moreover, desensitization of the kinase C pathway by prolonged exposure to phorbol esters abolished the induction of c-*myc* but did not affect PDGF-mediated mitogenesis.[147] These important experiments directly prove that other mechanisms than those leading to oncogene activation must be involved in PDGF action. PDGF receptor is definitely the first target in PDGF action, since only cells that express the receptor respond to PDGF. However, even chronic exogenous PDGF treatment by itself does not transform cells.[149] Huang et al.[149] found that antisera to PDGF only partially inhibited growth but did not revert transformation of certain SSV-transformed cell lines which suggests intracellular actin of v-*sis* product. These data were supported by Keating and Williams[150] who found that, in v-*sis* transformed cells, the majority of PDGF receptor activation occurs in intracellular compartments before receptor maturation and, therefore, before the receptors reach the cell surface. Existence of intracellular activation of PDGF receptors, however, is denied by other authors.[151]

## 3. NGF

After 40 years of extensive studies on the first discovered growth factor, nerve growth factor (NGF), the molecular mechanism of this growth factor action remains unknown.[152,153] Three groups of cells are targets for NGF: (1) neural crest derivatives; (2) central nervous system; and (3) cells of non-neural origin, such as mast cells.[152-156] NGF exerts different effects in particular cell types.[154,155]

NGF is essential for the maturation of sympathetic neurons and some sensory neurons,[152-161] but does not act as a mitogenic factor for embryonic sympathoadrenal progenitors.[162,163] In contrast, NGF exhibits mitogenic activity in early postnatal adrenal chromaffin cells.[164-166] NGF receptors were also found on neural crest-derived tumors, i.e., melanoma[31,167,168] and pheochromocytoma.[169,170] In rat pheochromocytoma cell line PC12, NGF induces differentiation without proliferation.[170] In melanoma cells, NGF inhibits cell division.[171-174] Recently we found NGF receptors on colorectal carcinoma and breast carcinoma cells.[171,175,176]

NGF is believed to recognize two types of the surface (plasma membrane) receptors: the low molecular weight ($M_r$ 75,000) receptor, which is well characterized and cloned in humans[32,33] and rats;[177] and the more recently identified, high molecular weight ($M_r$ 140,000) receptor.[34-36] The 140,000-$M_r$ receptor represents a product of the *trk* proto-oncongene (p140$^{trk}$). Each of the receptors binds NGF with low affinity, while the heterodimer of both receptors binds NGF with high affinity.[37] Klein et al.[35] found that p140$^{trk}$ alone may also generate high affinity receptors.

The *trk* gene is expressed predominantly in sensory neurons of spinal ganglia and in the portion of sensory neurons of cranial ganglia that originates from the neural crest.[178,179] NGF specifically stimulates tyrosine autophosphorylation of p140$^{trk}$.[34,178-180] Antibodies against p140 immunoprecipitate NGF crosslinked to the p140,[34,35] which proves that interaction of NGF with p140 occurs in intact cells. Complex p140-p75 seems to be specifically involved in binding of NGF,[179] in contrast to the low molecular weight NGF receptor ($M_r$ 75 to 80 kDa), which binds NGF as well as other members of the neurotrophin family, such as brain-derived neurotrophin factor (BDNF) and neurotrophin-3 (NT-3) with comparably low affinity (kDa of $10^{-9}$ $M$).[181] Another transmembrane tyrosine kinase protein (*trk* B) closely related in structure to p140[*trk*], and also expressed in the nervous system, binds BDNF and NT-3, but does not bind NGF.[182,183] The recently characterized *trk* C represents a specific receptor for neurotrophin-3.[184]

NGF treatment leads to a large number of metabolic alterations in responsive neurons, including specific induction of neurotransmitter biosynthetic enzymes such as tyrosine hydroxylase and dopamine hydroxylase,[185] choline acetyltransferase,[186,187] and phenylethanolamine-$N$-methyltransferase,[188] as well as other enzymes such as ornithine decarboxylase.[189,190] NGF also greatly enhances glucose and uridine uptake but does not activate $Na^+/H^+$ exchange.[191,192] NGF induces phosphorylation of cytoplasmic and nuclear proteins.[194,195] NGF has been shown to induce the expression of proto-oncogene c-*fos* in adrenal pheochromocytoma PC12 cells.[45,46,193-195] Calcium-binding proteins[196] and filament proteins[197] are also activated in response to NGF. Several second messengers (cAMP and diacylglycerol acting through protein kinase) were also proposed to be involved in NGF action.[1] However, until now there is no answer for the question of how NGF exerts different effects in different cell types, i.e., what the molecular mechanism of stimulation or inhibition of cell proliferation by NGF and/or activation of differentiation may be.

## II. NUCLEAR ACCUMULATION OF GROWTH FACTORS — REVOLUTIONARY DISCOVERY OR EXPERIMENTAL ARTIFACT?

Internalization through the cell surface receptor-mediated endocytosis and intracytoplasmic degradation are two dogmatic steps in growth factors action. Several laboratories have concentrated specifically on intracellular steps of growth factors degradation, and documenting that internalization is followed by complete degradation of the growth factor.[198-204] Highly controversial data, obtained independently in several laboratories, indicate that a fraction of internalized factors in a nondegraded form reaches the cell nucleus. The following growth factors were detected in the nucleus of target cells: NGF,[205-214] brain-derived neurotrophic factor (BDNF),[215] EGF,[216-221] PDGF,[222-225] fibroblast growth factor (FGF),[226-228] insulin,[229-235] insulin-like growth factor I (IGF-I),[236] interleukin 1 (IL-1),[237,238] angiotensin II,[239-242] vasoactive intestinal peptide,[243] and prolactin.[244]

### A. NGF

Nuclear interaction of NGF was reported for the first time by Andres et al.[205] Two classes of NGF receptors were described in embryonic dorsal root neurons: one class localized in plasma membranes and the other in the cell nucleus. Plasma membrane receptors could be solubilized by Triton X-100 and showed nonsaturable binding of NGF; plasma membrane tightly bound to the chromatin nuclear receptor for NGF was not extracted by Triton X-100 and showed saturable binding of NGF.[205]

Yanker and Shooter[206] incubated PC12 cells with [125]I-NGF and found that NGF was detectable in the nucleus after 20 min of incubation and continued to accumulate in a linear fashion during several hours of incubation. After 17 h at 37°C, 60% of NGF bound to the cell was in the nucleus. The receptors for NGF were localized in the chromatin. Electrophoretic mobility of the nuclear NGF was the same as that of the native NGF.[206]

Perinuclear and intranuclear localization of NGF in PC12 cells was confirmed by Marchisio et al.[207] using immunofluorescence staining and autoradiography. Nuclear accumulation of NGF was observed within the first hours of incubation. Association of NGF with nucleolus was also observed.[207] Marchisio et al.[207] suggested that NGF remains in contact with a pool of tubulin or actin molecules. Interaction of NGF with tubulin and actin was also described by other authors.[208] Recently, Piovo et al.[209] localized NGF in the nuclear membrane of rat basalic neurons.

The most extensive studies on nuclear accumulation of NGF in tumor cell lines have been performed by our laboratory.[171-175,210-214] We have identified the nuclear receptor for NGF using mAb to the NGF cell surface receptor.[171,174,176,210,212,214] According to our studies, binding of NGF to the cell surface receptor activates cell growth, while binding to the nuclear receptor inhibits rRNA synthesis and leads to tumor cell growth inhibition.[171-174,176,211]

## B. BDNF

So far, there is a single report[215] on nuclear localization of BDNF in neurons of rat hippocampal and cortical areas, which produce BDNF. Cytoplasmic accumulation was also observed in cholinergic neurons which do not synthesize BDNF. The authors suggest that one form of BDNF enters the nucleus of the producer-cell and may directly influence transcription, while another fraction of BDNF is secreted and is taken up by cholinergic neurons.[215]

## C. EGF

Pioneer experiments leading to discovery of the nuclear accumulation of EGF were performed by Gospodarowicz's laboratory and published in 1980.[216,217] The authors described interesting observations concerning the effect of EGF on changes of the chromatin structure in GH3 cells in the way that it increased binding of the bacterial RNA polymerase.[216] Further studies of these investigators resulted in the detection of EGF in the nucleus of cultured rat pituitary cells[217] and in bovine corneal endothelial and granulosa cells.[218] In the experimental system described in both papers,[217,218] EGF accumulated in the nucleus when lysosomal degradation was inhibited by chloroquine.

Recently Murawsky et al.[219] described the nuclear uptake of EGF in the presence or absence of chloroquine, in primary culture of rat hepatocytes.

Using different tumor cell lines, such as epidermoid carcinoma, colorectal carcinoma, breasts carcinoma, and normal fibroblasts, our laboratory detected EGF in the chromatin in the absence of inhibitors of lysosomal degradation.[175,220] Chromatin-bound EGF was nondegraded after 24 h of incubation and bound to a single *Eco*RI fragment of the chromatin.[220] We identified the nuclear receptor for EGF, using the mAb against the cell surface receptor.[220] In contrast to NGF or PDGF, EGF does not affect rRNA synthesis, which makes it likely that unique genes are regulated directly by chromatin bound EGF.[172] These results are described in detail in Section III of this chapter.

### D. PDGF

Nuclear translocation of the [125]I-PDGF, internalized by normal fibroblasts or by cancer cells (A,B heterodimer), was demonstrated by our laboratory in 1986,[175] followed by indication that translocation of PDGF to the chromatin of melanoma cells modulates DNAase II sensitivity of the chromatin[175] and activates rRNA synthesis, which results in increased cell proliferation.[177] We also found that NGF, after binding to the chromatin, antagonizes the effect of PDGF, i.e., inhibits rRNA synthesis.[172] Our results are described in Section III of this chapter.

Using alternative methods (immunogold labeling of cryosections), van den Eijnden-van Raaij and collaborators[222] detected PDGF in the nucleus of fibroblasts. In contrast to the nuclear accumulation of the taken-up by cell from the culture medium PDGF, PDGF produced by neuroblastoma cells or v-*sis* product in SSV-infected cells did not accumulate in the nucleus.[222] Different data were presented by Yeh and collaborators[223] who demonstrated by immunofluorescence staining, the nuclear (chromatin) localization of v-*sis* protein(s) in cells transformed with SSV. The last observation was partially supported by Lee et al.[224] who found that v-*sis* protein has a nuclear transport signal, localized within amino acid residues 237 to 255. Using a v-*sis* mutant, lacking N-terminal signal sequences determining transport of the nascent protein across the endoplasmic reticulum, which is common for all secretory proteins, Lee et al.[224] indicated nuclear and nucleolar localization of v-*sis*. More recent studies performed by Pierce et al.[225] indicated the presence in SSV-infected cells of two nuclear proteins, 65 kDa and 66 kDa, crossreactive with antibodies against PDGF or v-*sis* product. The third PDGF-like protein (44 kDa) was detected in both non-infected and infected cells.[225] Whether all three proteins represent products of an alternatively spliced v-*sis* or other PDGF-like proteins was not established.

### E. FGF

The most advanced studies on nuclear translocation of internalized FGF were obtained in Bouche's laboratory.[226,227] Convincing data indicate that FGF accumulates in the nucleus (nucleolus), specifically in the G1 phase, and stimulates transcription of ribosomal gene. Recently, Tessler et al.[228] described nuclear accumulation of FGF in cells transfected with bFGF genes (producing FGF). Data on nuclear uptake of FGF are discussed by Bouche et al. in Chapter 2 of this book.

### F. INSULIN

Nuclear uptake of insulin was first demonstrated by Lee and Williams.[229] The investigators infused radiodinated insulin into the veins of the isolated rat livers and next prepared subcellular fractions; insulin was associated with the nuclear, mitochondrial, and microsomal fractions. Sixteen years later, Arguilla[230] detected insulin in rat liver nuclei. Goldfine et al.[231] demonstrated uptake and nuclear binding of [125]I-insulin by lymphocytes. Uptake to [125]I-insulin reached maximum within 2 min of incubation; nuclei accumulated 15 to 20% of the total cellular radioactivity.[231] Vigneri et al.[232] described nuclear envelope as the major target site for insulin in rat liver nuclei. Recent data from Jarett's laboratory[233,234] suggest that insulin appears in the nucleus in the complex with the cell surface receptor.

Our laboratory found that [125]I-insulin is effectively internalized by several tumor cell lines and that a significant fraction of cell-bound insulin reaches the nucleus and binds to a 45,000 $M_r$ protein which seems to represent nuclear receptor.[235] Our data are discussed in Section III of this chapter.

## G. IGF-I

Soler et al.[236] used electron microscopy to detect IGF-I in the nucleus of the epithelial cells from chicken embryonic lens. The cells, after differentiation into fiber cells, lost the ability to accumulate IGF-I in the nucleus, which, according to the authors,[236] may relate to specificity of growth factor action in particular cell types.

## H. IL-I

IL-I, after binding to the cell surface receptor is extensively internalized. Internalization of IL-2 is required for its biological activity.[237] Grenfell et al.[238] found that internalized IL-1 enters the nucleus and may be extracted from the nucleus in a nondegraded form. IGF-I binds also to isolated nuclei, exhibiting a single high-affinity binding site (Kd 17 p$M$) and 79 binding sites per nucleus.[238]

## I. ANGIOTENSIN II

Several papers from Re's laboratory[239-242] are concentrated on the nuclear receptors for the protein hormone — angiotensin. The experiments were performed in a cell free system; angiotensin II penetrated the nuclei of rat liver which resulted in higher chromatin solubility. The authors concluded that angiotensin II affects chromatin structure, making it more accessible for endonuclease attack.[240,241] Action of angiotensin II at the intracellular level is discussed by Re in Chapter 3.

## J. VASOACTIVE INTESTINAL PEPTIDE

Omary and Kagnoff[243] described nuclear localization of the vasoactive intestinal peptide and also identified nuclear (chromatin) receptors for this peptide.

## K. PROLACTIN

Clevenger et al.[244] described nuclear translocation of prolactin in IL-2 stimulated T cells and concanavalin A stimulated splenocytes. Nuclear translocation of prolactin was inhibited by antiserum to prolactin which was added exogenously to the medium.

## L. CONCLUSIONS

Briefly summarized above, reports on nuclear accumulation of very different growth factors and peptide hormones suggest that nuclear translocation represents a general pathway in these molecules' action. Common to most of the reports is the observation that binding of nondegraded growth factors occurs to the nuclear receptors in a saturable and highly specific way.

# III. INTERNALIZATION AND NUCLEAR TRANSLOCATION OF GROWTH FACTORS — DIRECT EFFECT OF NGF ON EXPRESSION OF RIBOSOMAL RNA

## A. INTRACELLULAR DISTRIBUTION OF RADIOACTIVELY-LABELED GROWTH FACTORS

### 1. Internalization at Optimal Growth Conditions: 37°C, pH 7

Nerve growth factor (NGF), epidermal growth factor (EGF), platelet-derived growth factor (PDGF), insulin-like growth factor I (IGF-I), and insulin were labeled with $^{125}I$ and incubated at 37°C with cell lines that express different levels of cell surface receptors.[175,220,235] All growth factors were internalized by cells that express specific cell surface receptors (Table 1), but not by control cells that do not express the appropriate receptors. Internalization of $^{125}I$-labeled growth factors was inhibited 75 to 95% by the corresponding unlabeled growth factors. Internalization was completely abolished when cells were exposed to $^{125}I$-growth factors at 0 to 4°C (not shown), suggesting that the growth factors are specifically taken up by cells by receptor-mediated endocytosis. In most of the cell lines tested, the internalized growth factors were localized in the cytoplasm and in the nucleus. Kinetics of internalization and the number of growth factor molecules translocated to the nucleus were specific for the given growth factor and particular cell line (Table 1). The ratio between the number of $^{125}I$-growth factor molecules localized in the chromatin and in the nucleus varied in particular cell lines. Screening of a few melanoma cell lines (Table 1A) indicated that there are differences in the intracellular distribution of $^{125}I$-NGF. For example, in HS294 melanoma cells, during the first 24 h of incubation, $^{125}I$-NGF accumulated mainly in the cytoplasm, while after 48 h of incubation, it was localized mainly in the nucleus. This redistribution of $^{125}I$-NGF from the cytoplasm to the nucleus occurred with only an insignificant increase of the total amount of internalized growth factor. Redistribution of intracellular $^{125}I$-NGF between 24 and 48 h of incubation was also observed in the A875 melanoma cell line, but not in the 451 Lu melanoma cell line, where the total amount of internalized $^{125}I$-NGF was lower. In the WM164 cell line, internalization of $^{125}I$-NGF was very low and $^{125}I$-NGF did not accumulate in the nucleus. Rapid internalization and high nuclear accumulation of $^{125}I$-NGF were observed in the SKBr 5 breast carcinoma cell line. Colorectal carcinoma SW707 internalized much lower amounts of $^{125}I$-NGF than breast carcinoma and most of the melanoma cell lines (1000 molecules in the nucleus and the same amount in the cytoplasm). The SW948 colorectal carcinoma cell line does not express the NGF cell surface receptor and

## TABLE 1
### Internalization and Intracellular Distribution of Particular Growth Factors in Different Tumor Cell Lines

### Table 1A. NGF

| Cell line | Expression of cell surface receptor | Cell fraction | $^{125}$I-NGF molecules per cell fraction[a] | | |
|---|---|---|---|---|---|
| | | | 1 h | 24 h | 48 h |
| *Melanoma* | | | | | |
| HS294 | + + +[b] | C | 29,684 | 39,100 | 7,950 |
| | | NM | 110 | 350 | 200 |
| | | N | 100 | 450 | 750 |
| | | Ch | 500 | 4,000 | 42,200 |
| A875 | + + + | C | 20,500 | 29,000 | 22,000 |
| | | NM | 70 | 850 | 300 |
| | | N | 50 | 150 | 100 |
| | | Ch | 450 | 2,550 | 8,900 |
| 451Lu | + + | C | 1,100 | 3,850 | 5,000 |
| | | NM | 180 | 380 | 200 |
| | | N | 25 | 30 | 70 |
| | | Ch | 990 | 1,000 | 3,200 |
| WM164 | + | C | 700 | 1,500 | 3,000 |
| | | NM | 5 | 10 | 10 |
| | | N | 10 | 20 | 20 |
| | | Ch | 5 | 150 | 100 |
| *Breast carcinoma* | | | | | |
| SkBr 5 | + + | C | | 7,100 | |
| | | NM | | 450 | |
| | | N | | 120 | |
| | | Ch | | 25,890 | |
| *Colorectal carcinoma* | | | | | |
| SW707 | + | C | 490 | 780 | 1,200 |
| | | NM | 60 | 75 | 80 |
| | | N | 20 | 20 | 25 |
| | | Ch | 395 | 770 | 1,000 |
| SW948 | — | C | 210 | 220 | 220 |
| | | NM | 10 | 10 | 10 |
| | | N | 10 | 10 | 15 |
| | | Ch | 70 | 80 | 75 |
| *Glioma* | | | | | |
| V87Mg | + + | C | 1,325 | 10,800 | 20,500 |
| | | NM | 40 | 20 | 30 |
| | | N | 200 | 250 | 810 |
| | | Ch | 250 | 160 | 455 |
| V373Mg | + + | C | 44,000 | 31,000 | |
| | | NM | 15 | 65 | |
| | | N | 200 | 390 | |

**TABLE 1 (continued)**
**Internalization and Intracellular Distribution of Particular**
**Growth Factors in Different Tumor Cell Lines**

**Table 1A. NGF**

| Cell line | Expression of cell surface receptor | Cell fraction | $^{125}$I-NGF molecules per cell fraction[a] | | |
|---|---|---|---|---|---|
| | | | 1 h | 24 h | 48 h |
| *Leukemic T cells* | | | | | |
| SupT1 | | C | 70,000[c] | 25,000[d] | 3,000[e] |
| | | NM | 50 | 20 | 0 |
| | | N | 1,000 | 30 | 0 |
| | | Ch | 10 | 0 | 0 |

**Table 1B. EGF**

| Cell line | Expression of cell surface receptor | Cell fraction | $^{125}$I-EGF molecules per cell fraction[a] | | |
|---|---|---|---|---|---|
| | | | 1 h | 24 h | 48 h |
| *Fibroblasts* | | | | | |
| W138 | +[b] | C | 25,500 | 28,900 | 30,000 |
| | | NM | 100 | 120 | 110 |
| | | N | 180 | 100 | 120 |
| | | Ch | 300 | 580 | 600 |
| *Colorectal carcinoma* | | | | | |
| SW948 | + + | C | 71,000 | 105,000 | 147,450 |
| | | NM | 500 | 700 | 650 |
| | | N | 1,000 | 5,800 | 700 |
| | | Ch | 1,500 | 4,630 | 7,200 |
| SW707 | + / − | C | 300 | 400 | 580 |
| | | NM | 20 | 15 | 10 |
| | | N | 10 | 10 | 10 |
| | | Ch | 5 | 180 | 320 |
| *Epidermoid carcinoma* | | | | | |
| A431 | + + + | C | 170,000 | 250,000 | 300,000 |
| | | NM | 1,200 | 890 | 750 |
| | | N | 2,100 | 1,000 | 800 |
| | | Ch | 2,100 | 5,500 | 6,000 |

[a]    Mean from three to seven experiments; SD = 5 to 12%.
[b]    + + + corresponds to $10^6$ receptor molecules on one cell; + + to $5 \times 10^4$ to $10^5$ receptor molecules; and + to $10^3$ to $10^4$ receptor molecules.
[c]    10-min incubation.
[d]    1-h incubation.
[e]    4-h incubation.
[f]    C = cytoplasm; NM = nuclear membrane; N = nucleoplasm; Ch = chromatin.

## TABLE 1 (continued)
### Internalization and Intracellular Distribution of Particular Growth Factors in Different Tumor Cell Lines

### Table 1C. PDGF

| Cell line | Expression of cell surface receptor | Cell fraction | $^{125}$I-PDGF molecules per cell fraction[a] | | |
|---|---|---|---|---|---|
| | | | 1 h | 24 h | 48 h |
| *Fibroblasts* | | | | | |
| W138 | +[b] | C | 1,600 | 1,100 | 1,250 |
| | | NM | 70 | 75 | 80 |
| | | N | 80 | 70 | 75 |
| | | Ch | 545 | 800 | 650 |
| *Melanoma* | | | | | |
| WM266-5 | + | C | 650 | 1,200 | 1,500 |
| | | NM | 40 | 50 | 150 |
| | | N | 30 | 85 | 110 |
| | | Ch | 650 | 1,400 | 1,400 |
| *Lung carcinoma* | | | | | |
| 1810 | + | C | 1,120 | 1,300 | 1,500 |
| | | NM | 50 | 30 | 40 |
| | | N | 100 | 100 | 80 |
| | | Ch | 650 | 600 | 400 |
| *Fibroblasts* | | | | | |
| AG1523 | + + + | C | 18,000 | 32,000 | |
| | | NM | 100 | 120 | |
| | | N | 800 | 750 | |
| | | Ch | 3,000 | 3,200 | |

did not internalize $^{125}$I-NGF. Of two glioma cell lines tested, the V87 Mg cell line accumulated NGF only in the cytoplasm, while another, the V373 Mg cell line, accumulated NGF in both the cytoplasm and the nucleus (Table 10). In melanoma, breast carcinoma, and colorectal carcinoma cells, both nuclear and cytoplasmic accumulation increased with the time of incubation; accumulation was much higher after 24 or 48 h of incubation than after 1 h. Different kinetics of internalization were observed in T lymphocytes, which rapidly internalized $^{125}$I-NGF during the first minutes of incubation without chromatin binding of $^{125}$I-NGF. During the second to fourth hour of incubation, NGF was rapidly degraded (Table 1). Since we did not identify the NGF receptor on lymphocytes, we cannot establish whether the NGF receptor or any other NGF receptor homologous molecules expressed on T lymphocytes participate in the process of internalization. The results indicate that nuclear translocation of $^{125}$I-NGF represents a phenomenon that occurs in most but not all cell types that internalize this growth factor. The number of $^{125}$I-NGF molecules taken up by the nucleus does not correlate with the number of molecules internalized and accumulated in the cytoplasm. Based on these observations, non-specific adsorption of $^{125}$I-NGF to the chromatin during cell fractionation is unlikely.

**TABLE 1 (continued)**
**Internalization and Intracellular Distribution of Particular**
**Growth Factors in Different Tumor Cell Lines**

**Table 1D. Insulin**

| Cell line | Cell fraction[f] | [125]I-Insulin molecules per cell fraction[a] | | |
|---|---|---|---|---|
| | | 1 h | 24 h | 48 h |
| *Colorectal carcinoma* | | | | |
| SW948 | C | 1,350 | 20,000 | |
| | NM | 890 | 850 | |
| | N | 900 | 2,300 | |
| | Ch | 3,000 | 37,200 | |
| SW707 | C | 300 | 4,000 | 9,800 |
| | NM | 5 | 620 | 600 |
| | N | 45 | 2,000 | 400 |
| | Ch | 100 | 2,900 | 3,100 |
| *Melanoma* | | | | |
| WM266-4 | C | 1,200 | 11,500 | |
| | NM | 100 | 450 | |
| | N | 200 | 400 | |
| | Ch | 950 | 5,950 | |

[a]  Mean from three to seven experiments; SD = 5 to 12%.
[b]  + + + corresponds to $10^6$ receptor molecules on one cell; + + to $5 \times 10^4$ to $10^5$ receptor molecules; and + to $10^3$ to $10^4$ receptor molecules.
[c]  10-min incubation.
[d]  1-h incubation.
[e]  4-h incubation.
[f]  C = cytoplasm; NM = nuclear membrane; N = nucleoplasm; Ch = chromatin.

In contrast to [125]I-NGF, accumulation of which in the nucleus reached 50 to 70% of the amount internalized by the cell growth factor, [125]I-EGF predominantly accumulated in the cytoplasm, while the amount of chromatin bound [125]I-EGF never exceeded 2 to 7% of the total internalized [125]I-EGF (Table 1B). Thus, the molecular weight, which in the case of EGF (7,000) is lower than that of NGF (26,000), does not represent a parameter which is critical in nuclear translocation of growth factors. Since the cells were incubated with [125]I-EGF in the absence of inhibitors of lysosomal degradation, the low percentage of chromatin-bound EGF is consistent with the results obtained by other laboratories.[219] Lysosomal degradation of NGF is therefore several-fold lower than that of EGF.

[125]I-PDGF (AB-heterodimer) accumulated in cytoplasm and the nucleus (Table 1C). In contrast to NGF and EGF, [125]I-PDGF was very rapidly translocated to the

nucleus and bound to the chromatin. After 1 h of incubation, chromatin was "saturated" with $^{125}$I-PDGF and after longer incubation (24 to 48 h), the number of chromatin-bound $^{125}$I-PDGF molecules did not increase.

$^{125}$I-insulin was effectively internalized by the colorectal carcinoma and melanoma cell lines tested (Table 1D). In general, after 24 h of incubation, approximately tenfold more $^{125}$I-insulin was internalized than after 1 h of incubation. The amount of chromatin-bound $^{125}$I-insulin after 24 h varied in particular cell lines from 40 to 60% of internalized $^{125}$I-insulin.

## 2. Factors that Modulate Internalization and Nuclear Translocation of Growth Factors

Intracellular uptake and distribution of growth factors in particular cell compartments are constant for the given cell line and the restricted growth conditions. The results are highly reproducible; however, there are several factors modulating both intracellular uptake and nuclear translocation. As an example, we show how the distribution of $^{125}$I-NGF is affected in different conditions of cell growth. Internalization of $^{125}$I-NGF (Table 2) and all other growth factors (not shown) was blocked by 85 to 95% at 0°C. Optimal uptake of NGF occurred at a pH of approximately 7 and was dramatically blocked at a pH of around 8 or 6 (Table 2). After cell preincubation for 24 h with unlabeled NGF, total uptake of NGF within the first hours of incubation increased by a factor of 5, particularly preincubation with NGF modulated nuclear accumulation of NGF, which after preincubation was 5 times higher in SW707 colorectal carcinoma cells, but 50 times higher in A875 melanoma cells.

TPA exerted a strong effect on intracellular distribution of $^{125}$I-NGF (Table 2). TPA in the concentration $10^{-8}$ to $10^{-7}$ increased chromatin binding of NGF from 42% to 30.4% of the total cell-bound NGF, without any changes of the total intracellular uptake.

The results clearly document that internalization of $^{125}$I-NGF is followed by nuclear uptake and chromatin binding. Nuclear translocation represents an active process modulated significantly by several factors. The amount of the $^{125}$I-NGF accumulated in the nucleus does not directly depend on the number of the molecules entering the cell. Data presented in the next chapter will indicate that the number of the nuclear (chromatin) receptor-molecules determines NGF binding to the chromatin. Low temperature abolishes total internalization. Higher or lower pH decreases both internalization and nuclear translocation. Unlabeled ligand (NGF) modulates both internalization and nuclear translocation, but predominantly stimulates chromatin binding. TPA represents a factor modulating only chromatin binding of NGF (Table 2). Thus two processes that are synchronized, but independent in nature, take place in the cell: uptake into the cell and nuclear translocation with the chromatin binding.

## 3. Binding of NGF to Non-Mitotic Chromatin

Cells of the breast carcinoma line SKBr 5 grow in the culture medium and do not adhere, unless they undergo mitosis. Based on this property, we incubated a

## TABLE 2
### Factors that Modulate Nuclear Translocation of Growth Factors, Based on the Example of NGF: Temperature, pH, NGF, Phorbol Esters (TPA)

| Cell line | Temperature (°C) | pH | NGF preincubation (10 ng/ml) | TPA concentration (M) | Time of incubation with 10 ng/ml $^{125}$I-NGF (h) | $^{125}$I-NGF molecules per cell[a] | | | |
|---|---|---|---|---|---|---|---|---|---|
| | | | | | | C[b] | N | NM | Ch |
| *Melanoma* | | | | | | | | | |
| A875 | 0 | 7.15 | — | — | 1 | 1,000 | 0 | 0 | 0 |
| | 37 | 7.15 | — | — | 1 | 5,500 | 70 | 10 | 300 |
| | 37 | 8.20 | — | — | 1 | 1,400 | 5 | 10 | 100 |
| | 37 | 6.50 | — | — | 1 | 1,500 | 50 | 10 | 180 |
| | 37 | 7.15 | 24 h | 0 | 1 | 13,250 | 400 | 175 | 12,200 |
| | 37 | 7.15 | — | — | 24 | 44,150 | 680 | 300 | 5,690 |
| | 37 | 7.15 | — | $1 \times 10^{-8}$ | 24 | 45,000 | 1,090 | 350 | 6,630 |
| | 37 | 7.15 | — | $5 \times 10^{-8}$ | 24 | 39,670 | 1,000 | 435 | 12,070 |
| | 37 | 7.15 | — | $1 \times 10^{-7}$ | 24 | 35,500 | 1,300 | 420 | 16,100 |
| *Colorectal carcinoma* | | | | | | | | | |
| SW707 | 0 | 7.15 | — | — | 1 | 50 | 0 | 0 | 0 |
| | 37 | 7.15 | — | — | 1 | 750 | 10 | 0 | 620 |
| | 37 | 7.15 | 24 h | — | 1 | 1,220 | 125 | 5 | 3,000 |
| | 37 | 8.20 | 24 h | — | 1 | 420 | 5 | 0 | 200 |
| *Breast carcinoma* | | | | | | | | | |
| SKBr 5 | 0 | 7.15 | — | — | 1 | 500 | 40 | 20 | 20 |
| | 37 | 7.15 | — | — | 1 | 1,200 | 100 | 40 | 3,800 |
| | 37 | 8.20 | — | — | 1 | 620 | 20 | 10 | 1,300 |
| | 37 | 6.75 | — | — | 1 | 525 | 30 | 5 | 1,800 |

[a] Data from three to five experiments; SD < 15%.

[b] C = cytoplasm; N = nucleoplasm; NM = nuclear membrane; Ch = chromatin.

**TABLE 3**
**Internalization and Intracellular Distribution of $^{125}$I-NGF in
Non-Mitotic and Mitotic SKBr 5 Breast Carcinoma Cells
(24 h Incubation)[a]**

| Non-mitotic | | | | Mitotic | | | |
|---|---|---|---|---|---|---|---|
| C[b] | N | NM | Ch | C | N | NM | Ch |
| 8,500 | 100 | 700 | 44,000 | 4,800 | 80 | 30 | 8,100 |

[a]   Data are means from three to five experiments; SD = 15%.
[b]   C = cytoplasm; N = nucleus; NM = nuclear membrane; Ch = chromatin.

whole population of SKBr 5 cells for 24 h, then separated non-mitotic cells and mitotic cells and tested intracellular distribution of NGF.[212] Chromatin of non-mitotic cells incorporated five times more $^{125}$I-NGF than that of mitotic cells, while the cytoplasm of non-mitotic cells incorporated only twice more (Table 3). Both populations express the same number of cell surface receptors, which implies that the chromatin receptor for NGF is specifically bound to non-mitotic chromosomes. In mitotic cells, $^{125}$I-NGF is not bound to the chromatin and undergoes rapid degradation. The results further confirm the specificity of NGF binding to the chromatin and the role of the nuclear receptor in stabilizing the pool of intracellular NGF.

## B. DETECTION OF THE NUCLEAR NGF USING IMMUNOFLUORESCENCE STAINING

To determine whether the nuclear translocation of $^{125}$I-NGF observed in the cell fractionation studies reflects the physiological action of internalized NGF, or instead represents an artifact of the cell fractionation, intracellular localization of NGF was tested by indirect immunofluorescence staining (Figure 1).

Three groups of cells were tested:

1.   Melanoma cell line WM164, which expresses a very low number of cell surface receptors and internalizes low amounts of $^{125}$I-NGF into the cytoplasm, but not into the nucleus[174] (Table 1)

2.   Melanoma cell line A875, which expresses a high number of cell surface receptors and extensively internalizes $^{125}$I-NGF into cytoplasm and nucleus (Table 1)[171]

3.   Colorectal carcinoma cell line SW707, which internalizes low amounts of $^{125}$I-NGF; 50% into the nucleus[171]

After 1 h incubation of melanoma A875 cells with NGF, cytoplasmic fluorescence was strong and predominant, although nuclear fluorescence was also detectable with significantly stronger staining of the nucleolus (Figure 1A). When NGF was bound to the particles of the colloidal gold (10 nm), fluorescence was restricted to the cytoplasm (Figure 1B).

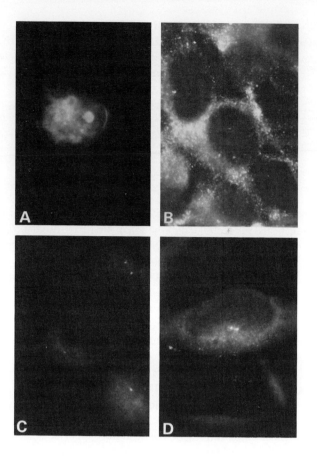

**FIGURE 1.**   Immunofluorescence detection of internalized NGF. Indirect immunofluorescence staining of A875 melanoma (A, B), WM164 melanoma (C, D), and SW707 colorectal carcinoma cells (E, F, G). Cells were incubated 1 h (A, B, C, E, G) or 24 h (D) with NGF (10 ng/ml) or colloidal gold (10 nm particles)-bound NGF (B), followed by incubation with anti-NGF rabbit serum and fluoresceine-conjugated sheep anti-rabbit IgG. In (G), SW707 cells were not incubated with NGF. Cytoplasm (C), nucleus (N), and nucleolus (NC) are shown by arrows. (Figures E, F, and G are from Rakowicz-Szulczynska, E. M., Reddy, U., Vorbrodt, A., Herlyn, D., and Koprowski, H., *Mol. Carcinogen.*, 2, 47, copyright © 1989. With permission of Wiley-Liss, division of John Wiley and Sons, Inc.)

In WM164 melanoma cells incubated 24 h with NGF, only a very weak fluorescence of the cytoplasm was detected. No fluorescence staining of the nucleus was visible (Figure 1C and D).

After a 30-min incubation of SW707 cells with NGF (10 ng/ml), the fluorescence was detected almost exclusively in the nucleus (Figure 1E). After a 24-h exposure to NGF, cells also showed fluorescence in the cytoplasm (Figure 1G). In control experiments, cells not exposed to NGF did not stain with rabbit anti-NGF serum (Figure 1F).

The results indicate that in intact SW707 and A875 cells, NGF specifically accumulates in the cell nucleus. The kinetics of fluorescence staining of SW707

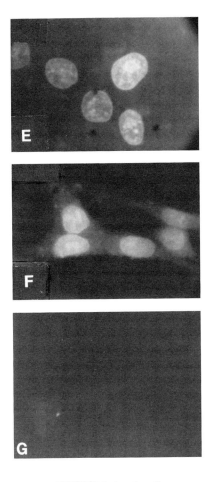

**FIGURE 1.** (continued)

cells suggest that NGF taken up by the cell is initially rapidly translocated to the cell nucleus, and, after saturating the nuclear receptor, later accumulates in the cytoplasm. These events are visible only in SW707 cells in which no more than 1500 molecules of NGF accumulate in the cell. In the melanoma A875 cells, in which more than 20,000 molecules penetrate the cell, strong fluorescence of the cytoplasm partially masks the nuclear accumulation of NGF. In contrast, in WM164 melanoma cells, NGF accumulates only in the cytoplasm.

Since both SW707 and WM164 cells internalized a similar number of [125]I-NGF molecules (1,500/cell) (Table 1), the lack of nuclear accumulation of NGF in WM164 cells indicates that a specific mechanism of nuclear accumulation of NGF must be present in SW707 cells. In Chapter 4, we will present experiments suggesting that a specific nuclear protein (receptor) expressed in SW707 and A875 cells, but not in WM164 cells, binds the NGF translocated to the nucleus.

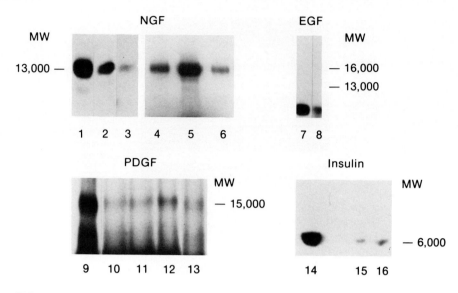

**FIGURE 2.** SDS-PAGE (10 to 15% polyacrylamide gel, 12-h autoradiographic exposure) of chromatin-bound $^{125}$I-growth factors after 24-h incubation with intact cells. Lane 1, free $^{125}$I-NGF; lane 2, $^{125}$I-NGF extracted from the chromatin of HS294 melanoma cells; lane 3, SW707 colorectal carcinoma; lane 4, glioma V373 Mg; lane 5, SKBr 5 breast carcinoma; lane 6, melanoma A875; lane 7, free $^{125}$I-EGF; lane 8, $^{125}$I-EGF extracted from SW948 colorectal carcinoma cell chromatin; lane 9, free $^{125}$I-PDGF; lane 10, $^{125}$I-PDGF extracted from the chromatin of SW707 colorectal carcinoma cells; lane 11, WM266-4 melanoma; lane 12, AG1523 lung fibroblasts; lane 13, 1810 lung tumor cells; lane 14, free $^{125}$I-insulin; lane 15, $^{125}$I-insulin extracted from the chromatin of WM266-4 melanoma cells; lane 16, $^{125}$I-insulin extracted from SW948 colorectal carcinoma cells. Electrophoresis according to Laemmli.[245]

## C. CHROMATIN BINDING OF NONDEGRADED GROWTH FACTORS

$^{125}$I-NGF, PDGF, EGF, and insulin, when extracted from the chromatin with 1% sodium dodecyl sulfate (SDS), showed the same electrophoretic mobility as free growth factors (Figure 2), which suggests that a fraction of internalized growth factors reaches the nucleus and binds to the chromatin in a nondegraded form.

Extraction of $^{125}$I-growth factor-bound chromatin (isolated from cells incubated with $^{125}$I-growth factor) with 0.35 $M$ NaCl and 2 $M$ NaCl, released only up to 35% of $^{125}$I-NGF, $^{125}$I-EGF, or $^{125}$I-PDGF (Table 4). Since 0.35 $M$ NaCl releases most of nonhistone proteins loosely bound to the chromatin, and 2 $M$ NaCl most of the tightly bound nonhistones and histones, we conclude that up to 65% of all three growth factors, NGF, EGF, and PDGF, bind very tightly to the residual chromatin fraction.[171,175,210] It was shown previously that the residual chromatin fraction represents a tissue-specific complex of DNA and regulatory nonhistone proteins.[246,247] To test whether $^{125}$I-growth factors bind to DNAse-sensitive, actively-transcribed chromatin regions, chromatin extracted from cells exposed for 1, 12, or 24 h to one of the tested growth factors was digested with DNAse II, until 12 to 20% of

## TABLE 4
### Presence of $^{125}$I-Growth Factors in Salt-Extracted Chromatin after 24 h Incubation of Intact Cells

| Chromatin treatment | Percentage of [$^{125}$I]-growth factor-bound[a] | | | |
|---|---|---|---|---|
| | $^{125}$I-NGF[b] | $^{125}$I-PDGF[c] | $^{125}$I-EGF[d] | $^{125}$I-Insulin[e] |
| Intact | 100 | 100 | 100 | 100 |
| 0.35 *M* NaCl | 85.5 ± 1.5 | 70 ± 3.0 | 75 ± 50 | 40 ± 10 |
| 2 *M* NaCl | 80 ± 1.5 | 65 ± 50 | 70 ± 50 | 35 ± 5 |

[a]　Mean ± SD from three experiments.
[b]　A875 melanoma cell line.
[c]　WM266 melanoma cell line.
[d,e]　SW948 colorectal carcinoma cell line.

DNAse II-sensitive sequences were digested.[171,175,210] When the chromatin originated from cells exposed for 1 h to $^{125}$I-NGF (Figure 3), $^{125}$I-EGF, or $^{125}$I-PDGF (not shown), digestion of approximately 12 to 13% of the DNA sequences released 50 to 70% of each of the growth factors tested. However, when the chromatin originated from cells exposed to 24 or 48 h of the growth factor, no $^{125}$I-NGF (or other growth factors) release was observed (Figure 3). These results suggest that growth factors bind to DNAse II-sensitive chromatin regions which, after ''saturation'' with the growth factor, become protected against DNAse II-digestion.

In order to test whether the chromatin-bound growth factors are randomly bound to DNAse II-sensitive chromatin regions, or instead are bound to specific DNA regions, chromatin was isolated from cells exposed for 24 h to $^{125}$I-growth factor and digested with *Eco*RI, *Bam*HI or *Hinc*II restriction nucleases. Digestion of SW948 colorectal carcinoma cell chromatin with *Eco*RI released a single DNA fragment bound to $^{125}$I-EGF[220] (Figure 4). Thus, $^{125}$I-EGF molecules that enter the nucleus interact with a very specific chromatin region. The results eliminate nonspecific, artificial attachment of $^{125}$I-EGF to the chromatin during cell fractionation. If $^{125}$I-EGF attached nonspecifically to the chromatin, then a smear of $^{125}$I-EGF bound randomly to several DNA fragment should have been observed. Digestion of $^{125}$I-insulin-bound chromatin from the same SW948 cell line with *Eco*RI[235] also released a single DNA fragment, but of an electrophoretic mobility four times lower than that of the DNA fragment bound to $^{125}$I-EGF (Figure 4). Digestion of the chromatin with *Hae*III released three $^{125}$I-insulin-bound fragments, and *Hinc*III released one fragment (Figure 4). $^{125}$I-NGF and $^{125}$I-PDGF were not released by chromatin digestion with any of the used restriction nucleases (*Eco*RI, *Hinc*II, *Hae*III, *Bam*HI), which suggests that DNA regions located near these growth factors' binding sites are either protected by nonhistone proteins, or by growth factors bound to the chromatin.

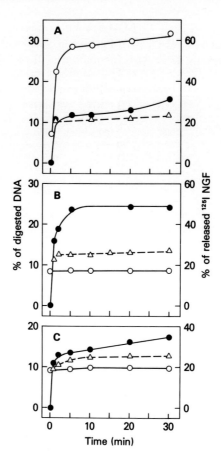

**FIGURE 3.** Release of $^{125}$I-NGF (○) from the DNAseII-digested chromatin isolated from HS294 melanoma cells exposed to $^{125}$I-NGF (10 ng/ml) for 1 h (A), 24 h (B), and 48 h (C). Percentage of the digested DNA sequences (●) and percentage of the digested $Mg^{2+}$-soluble, actively transcribed sequences (△) are shown. The conditions of the experiments were described.[175]

## D. IDENTIFICATION OF NUCLEAR RECEPTORS FOR GROWTH FACTORS

Binding of $^{125}$I-growth factors to specific chromatin regions (DNA fragments) (Figure 4) and modulating DNAseII sensitivity of certain chromatin regions (Figure 3) strongly suggested that growth factors must recognize specific chromatin targets which could be represented by specific DNA sequences or by chromatin proteins. $^{125}$I-NGF, EGF, PDGF, and insulin were tested for the ability to bind to the fragments of the naked DNA, using filter-binding assays or a DNA-affinity column. No direct binding of $^{125}$I-growth factors to DNA was observed. To eliminate the possibility that single growth factor molecules bind to unique sequences of DNA and therefore cannot be detected by measuring the radioactivity of $^{125}$I-growth factor bound to

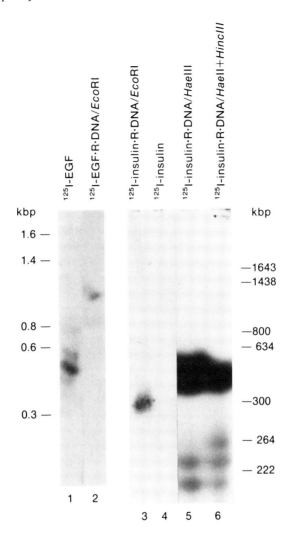

**FIGURE 4.** Electrophoretic detection of free [125]I-EGF (lane 1) and [125]I-EGF bound to an *Eco*RI-DNA fragment during 24 h of incubation of SW948 cells (lane 2). Chromatin from cells incubated for 2 h with [125]I-EGF was digested with *Eco*RI, and the supernatant was analyzed in 4% polyacrylamide gel containing 50 m$M$ Tris, 384 m$M$ glycine, and 2 m$M$ EDTA, pH 8.3. Gels were dried and autoradiographed. Free [125]I-EGF and DNA-bound [125]I-EGF show different electrophoretic mobility (lanes 1 and 2). In the same procedure, insulin binds to a single *Eco*RI-chromatin fragment (lane 3), three *Hae*III fragments (lane 5), and one *Hinc*II fragment (lane 6). Free [125]I-insulin (lane 4) migrates out of the gel. R stands for chromatin receptor which binds the growth factor to the specific restriction fragment.

DNA, DNA-[125]I-growth factor complexes potentially remaining on the nitrocellulose filter were cloned in PUC8. No positive clones were obtained, which further eliminates the possibility of direct binding of NGF, EGF, PDGF, and insulin to the naked DNA of the target cells. Instead, all growth factors tested bound efficiently to the native chromatin. We have found that binding of [125]I-NGF or [125]I-EGF to the chromatin isolated from target cells may be efficiently inhibited by an unlabeled growth factor, as well as by the mAb developed against the appropriate cell surface receptor.[175] The experiments suggested that a molecule of an epitopic homology to the cell surface receptor may be expressed in the chromatin of target cells. Since we have indicated in Table 2 that growth factor-binding "sites" in the chromatin are very tightly bound to DNA and are not extracted with 2 $M$ NaCl, it was unlikely that we would be able to isolate the growth factor-binding chromatin proteins without the use of denaturing agents, such as SDS or Triton X-100. To eliminate the denaturing conditions needed to dissociate proteins from DNA, we have developed a method for immunoprecipitation of the chromatin proteins bound to DNA fragments.[210] In this method, chromatin is isolated from cells (not exposed to the growth factor) and digested with *Eco*RI or another restriction nuclease. The DNA-protein complexes released from the chromatin by the restriction nuclease are treated with mAb developed originally against the cell surface receptor of the growth factor tested. The mAb binds to the chromatin protein which expresses an epitope homologous to that expressed by the cell surface receptor. In the consequence of the complexes containing all three components, mAb — chromatin receptor — DNA, fragments are precipitated and may be removed from the medium by attachment to *Staphyloccus aureus* (or protein A-agarose beads). After treatment with SDS, the receptor dissociates from the mAb and DNA and may be analyzed by SDS-polyacrylamide gel electrophoresis (PAGE).[210] Since usually the chromatin receptors are expressed in very low quantities and are undetectable by Coomassie blue staining, chromatin is isolated from cells labeled with [[35]S]methionine. Using the procedure described, we were able to identify a family of nuclear proteins which exhibit different molecular weights than the cell surface receptors for NGF and EGF, but must express the same epitopes which are recognized by the appropriate mAbs developed originally against the cell surface receptors.[171,174,210,212,214,220] We named these proteins chromatin receptors for growth factors, although it is still unknown whether there is a structural, or only conformational homology between the cell surface receptors and the growth factor-binding nuclear protein.

## 1. NGF Receptors

### a. 230,000-$M_r$ Chromatin Receptor

mAb 20.4 and mAb 82.11 developed against NGF cell surface receptor[31] immunoprecipitate both the cell surface receptors[32,33,168] and the chromatin receptors from a broad range of cell lines tested (melanoma cells, normal melanocytes, glioma, breast carcinoma, and colorectal carcinoma).[171,174,210-212,214,220] The chromatin receptors for NGF immunoprecipitated from melanoma cell lines (Figure 5, lanes 3 to 5), and glioma cell lines (Figure 5, lane 7) exhibit high molecular weight ($M_r$

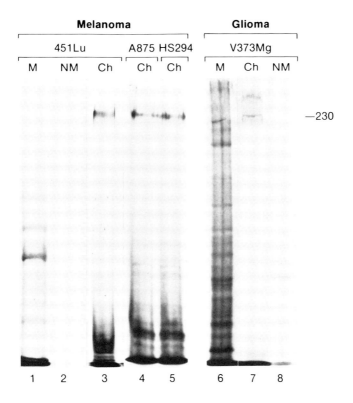

**FIGURE 5.** SDS PAGE (7.5% polyacrylamide gel) and autoradiographic detection of plasma membrane (M), nuclear membrane (NM), and chromatin proteins immunoprecipitated by mAb ME 20.4 against NGF receptor, from different melanoma or glioma cells, labeled with [$^{35}$S]methionine. A 70,000-$M_r$ plasma membrane receptor was immunoprecipitated from melanoma cells (lane 1) and a 140,000-$M_r$ receptor from glioma cells (lane 6). A 230,000-$M_r$ chromatin protein was immunoprecipitated from all cell lines (lanes 3 to 5, 7). In glioma cells, a 280,000-$M_r$ protein band co-immunoprecipitated with the 230,000-$M_r$ band (lane 7). No protein was immunoprecipitated from the nuclear membrane fraction (lanes 2 and 8).

230,000). In glioma cells, in addition to the 230,000 $M_r$ receptor, a 280,000-$M_r$ receptor-form was also visible (lane 7). No protein was immunoprecipitated by mAb 20.4 from the chromatin "saturated" with NGF, which proves that the 230,000 $M_r$ protein detected by anti-NGF receptor mAb represents the nuclear (chromatin) receptor for NGF. The cell surface receptor for NGF exhibits a low molecular weight in melanoma cells (75,000) (Figure 5, lane 1), but a high molecular weight (140,000) in glioma cells (Figure 5, lane 6). Chao et al.[32] indicated that the melanoma cell 75,000-$M_r$ cell surface receptor is a typical low affinity receptor. The 140,000 $M_r$ receptor detected in glioma cells (Figure 5, lane 6) is likely to represent the high affinity receptor for NGF which was characterized as the product of the *trk* protooncogene. Alternatively, it may represent a different molecular form of the low-affinity receptor.

The 230,000-$M_r$ chromatin protein (Figure 5, lanes 3 to 5) was undetectable in the cell membrane fraction (Figure 5, lane 2), and the 70,000-$M_r$ cell surface receptor was undetectable in the chromatin fraction, which proves that mAb ME 20.4 immunoprecipitates two proteins belonging to different cellular compartments. In order to eliminate the possibility that the chromatin protein represents an aggregated form of the 70,000-$M_r$ plasma membrane receptor (which during cell fractionation might have attached to the nuclear membranes and next to the chromatin), the nuclear membrane fraction was also immunoprecipitated with mAb ME 20.4. Neither the 230,000-$M_r$ chromatin protein nor the 70,000-$M_r$ membrane protein were immunoprecipitated from the nuclear membrane fraction of melanoma or glioma cells (Figure 5, lanes 2 and 8), which proves that the nuclei we used were free from cytoplasmic contaminations.

In further studies we concentrated on the 230,000-$M_r$ protein abundantly expressed in the chromatin of the melanoma 451 Lu.[214] The 230,000-$M_r$ diffuse band was immunoprecipitated from 451 Lu melanoma cells not exposed (Figure 6, lane 1) or exposed (Figure 6, lanes 2 and 3) to NGF (10 ng/ml). After a 1-week exposure of cells to NGF, the 230,000-$M_r$ band was much stronger, which suggested that NGF induced expression of this protein. When the cells were exposed to NGF for 10 to 24 h, in addition to the 230,000-$M_r$ protein, a 90,000-$M_r$ protein appeared (Figure 6, lane 3). We suggest that the 90,000-$M_r$ protein may represent a subunit of the 230,000-$M_r$ receptor, separated from the larger subunit after ligand (NGF) binding. Experiments described in later chapters strongly support this hypothesis. However, from the data presented in Figure 6, we cannot eliminate the possibility that the 90,000-$M_r$ protein band represents a degradation product of the 230,000-$M_r$ protein. Alternatively, the 90,000-$M_r$ band may represent a chromatin protein induced by NGF and bound to the same restriction fragment that the chromatin receptor binds.

The diffused shape of the immunoprecipitated chromatin receptor suggested that the protein may be glycosylated. The 230,000-$M_r$ protein fraction immunoprecipitated from the chromatin of melanoma cells by mAb ME 20.4 was electrophoretically separated in a 7.5% one-dimensional gel, transferred onto the nitrocellulose filter, and incubated with one of the three [125]I-labeled lectins: ConA, WGA (Figure 7), or lectin from *V. villosa* (not shown).[214] The reaction with each of the tested lectins was positive, which suggests that the 230,000-$M_r$ chromatin protein contains a heterogenous sugar component that probably consists of α-D-glucose and/or α-D-mannose (recognized by ConA), N-acetyl-β-D-glucosamine (recognized by WGA) and α-D-fucose and/or D-galactose and/or α-lactose recognized by the lectin from *V. villosa*.

After reaction with ConA, the 230,000-$M_r$ protein band showed two tightly spaced components with a molecular weight similar to the molecular weight of protein bands observed in the two-dimensional gel of the immunoprecipitate (Figure 8). It seems that only the higher molecular weight band reacted with WGA and the lectin from *V. villosa*. Two additional bands of lower molecular weight (approximately 90,000 and 80,000) were also detected by ConA. It is likely that the 90,000-

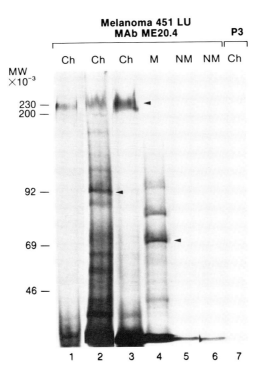

**FIGURE 6.** One-dimensional gel electrophoresis and autoradiographic detection of the cell surface and the chromatin receptor for NGF. [$^{35}$S]methionine-labeled chromatin proteins immunoprecipitated by mAb ME 20.4 (against plasma membrane NGF receptor) from chromatin of 451 Lu melanoma cells not exposed to NGF (lane 1), exposed to NGF (10 ng/ml) for 24 h (lane 2), or for 1 week (lane 3) were separated in 7.5% polyacrylamide gel with 0.1% SDS. Plasma membranes (lane 4) and nuclear membranes (lane 5) were immunoprecipitated with the same mAb ME 20.4 as controls for the purity of the chromatin fraction used for immunoprecipitation. A 70,000-$M_r$ major band of the plasma membrane receptor, followed by two higher molecular weight bands (75,000 and 90,000), was immunoprecipitated from plasma membranes and a 55,000-$M_r$ weak band from nuclear membrane fraction. The 55,000-$M_r$ nuclear membrane protein attaches to *S. aureus* also in the absence of mAb ME 20.4 (lane 6).

$M_r$ protein band corresponds to the 90,000-$M_r$ protein which dissociates from the 230,000-$M_r$ protein in the presence of NGF (Figure 6, lane 2). Alternatively, these bands may represent degradation products of the 230,000-$M_r$ protein or unrelated proteins which bind to the same *Eco*RI fragment and co-immunoprecipitate with the 230,000-$M_r$ protein.

Two-dimensional gel electrophoresis of the protein fraction (immunoprecipitated from the chromatin with mAb ME 20.4 and seen as a single, 230,000-$M_r$ protein-band in one-dimensional electrophoretic analysis) revealed a major 230,000-$M_r$ component in the region corresponding to a pI of approximately 6.2 and three minor components of $M_r$ 210,000 at a pI of 6.2, and $M_r$ 230,000 and 210,000 at a pI of 5.5[214] (Figure 8).

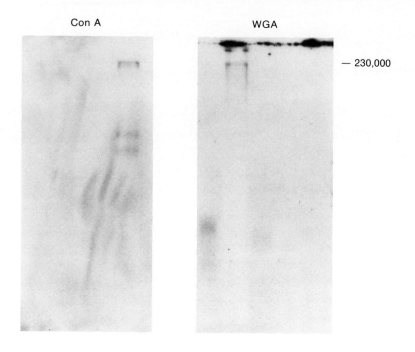

**FIGURE 7.**   Lectin binding by the 230,000-$M_r$ chromatin receptor. The chromatin receptor was immunoprecipitated from 451Lu melanoma cell chromatin with mAb ME 20.4, separated in 7.5% polyacrylamide gel, transferred onto nitrocellulose filter, and incubated with [125]I-ConA (binds to α-D-mannose and α-D-glucose or [125]I-WGA (binds to N-acetyl-β-D-glucosamine).

The presence of different subfractions in two-dimensional gel electrophoresis and of the diffuse single 230,000-$M_r$ band in one-dimensional electrophoresis seems to be due to the high and variable glycosylation of this protein.

The high molecular weight protein(s) immunoprecipitated by mAb ME 20.4 from [35S]methionine-labeled chromatin of 451 Lu were undetectable on the autoradiogram of total chromatin proteins separated by two-dimensional electrophoresis (Figure 9). When the cells were exposed for 10 d to NGF, mainly quantitative differences in the composition of several chromatin proteins were observed[214] (Figure 9). One protein, $M_r$ 230,000, isoelectric point 5.8, was detected only on the autoradiogram of cells exposed to NGF, but was undetectable in cells not exposed to NGF. Since the molecular weights of the protein induced by NGF corresponds to the $M_r$ (230,000) of the NGF chromatin receptor, it is likely that the chromatin receptor that is expressed in extremely low quantities became visualized among the total chromatin protein, after stimulation with NGF. Since neither mAb ME 20.4 nor NGF are able to bind to the denatured form of the chromatin receptor, we cannot verify this possibility by Western blotting.

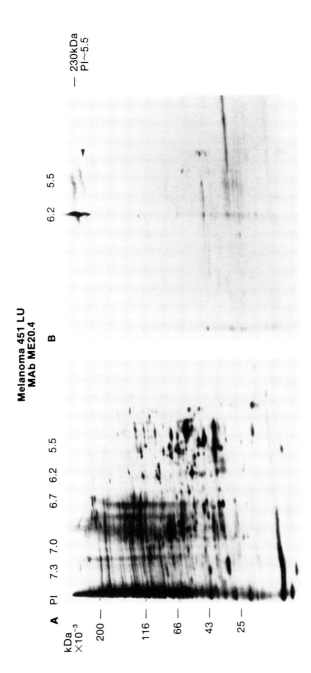

**FIGURE 8.** Two-dimensional gel electrophoresis of chromatin proteins and NGF chromatin receptor. [$^{35}$S]methionine-labeled chromatin proteins (A) and chromatin receptor immunoprecipitated with mAb ME 20.4 (B) were analyzed by isoelectrophoresis in one dimension (pH 2 to 8), and 5 to 15% SDS-gel electrophoresis in the second dimension. The major band of the chromatin receptor exhibits a $M_r$ of 230,000 and pI of 6.2; the three minor bands are 210,000 $M_r$, pI 6.2: 230,000 $M_r$, pI 5.5; and 210,000 $M_r$, pI 5.5.

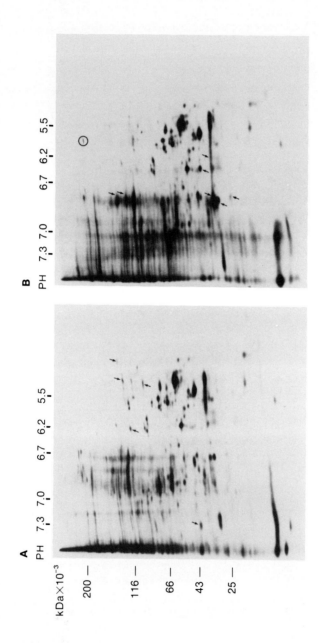

**FIGURE 9.** Effect of NGF on synthesis of chromatin proteins. Chromatin proteins were isolated from 451Lu melanoma cells incubated 18 h with [$^{35}$S]methionine in the absence (A) or presence (B) of NGF (10 ng/ml) and separated by two-dimensional gel electrophoresis. (Autoradiographic detection after 24 h of exposure.)

### b. Amino Acid Analysis of the 230,000-$M_r$ Chromatin Receptor

The 230,000-$M_r$ protein, immunoprecipitated by mAb ME 20.4 and separated in one-dimensional electrophoresis, was electroeluted from the gel and subjected to amino acid analysis. In order to eliminate the possibility that the chromatin receptor represents an aggregated form of the cell surface receptor, the amino acid composition of the chromatin receptor was compared with the amino acid composition of the cell surface receptor (Johnson et al., 1986) (Table 5). Approximately 28 residues of methionine, and a very low level of cysteine, were detected in the chromatin receptor. In contrast, the cell surface receptor contains more cysteine, but much less methionine. Compared to the surface receptor, the chromatin receptor contains several times more histidine, phenylalanine, and lysine, but only about 25% as much serine. Asparagine/aspartic acid and glutamine/glutamic acid residues represent in total more than 20% of amino acid residues in the chromatin receptor. Although we cannot distinguish between the acidic amino acid and the amid of these amino acids, we can expect that the protein contains a substantial number of acidic amino acids which are typical for the nonhistone chromatin protein. The presence of positively charged lysine and arginine suggests that the protein can potentially interact with DNA and acidic nonhistone proteins. NGF chromatin receptor is currently being microsequenced.

In contrast to the high molecular weight (230,000-$M_r$) chromatin receptor expressed by melanoma and glioma cells and described above, two other medium and low molecular weight receptor-species have been immunoprecipitated with mAb ME 20.4 and mAb 82.11 from breast carcinoma (Figure 10) and colorectal carcinoma cells (Figure 11; see below).

### c. 90,000-$M_r$ Chromatin Receptor

Breast carcinoma cell line SKBr5, which internalizes [125]I-NGF more efficiently than melanoma cell lines (Table 1), was found to express one type of the mAb ME 20.4-precipitable cell surface receptor ($M_r$ approximately 80,000) (Figure 10A, lanes 3 and 4).[212] Two receptor species were immunoprecipitated from the chromatin of breast carcinoma cells, the major protein of the $M_r$ 90,000 and the minor protein of the $M_r$ 200,000 (Figure 10A, lanes 1 and 2; Figure 10B, lanes 1 to 4). NGF added to the cell culture medium of SKBr 5 cells stimulated significant expression of the 200,000-$M_r$ chromatin protein, and to a lesser degree the 90,000-$M_r$ chromatin receptor (Figure 10A, lane 2; Figure 10B, lanes 2 and 4). Expression of the 80,000-$M_r$ cell surface receptor was also slightly stimulated by NGF (Figure 10A, lane 4). The 90,000-$M_r$ chromatin protein was the only receptor purified from the chromatin of SKBr 5 cell by affinity chromatography on mAb ME 20.4 (Figure 10C).

Pre-exposure of the chromatin to NGF abolished binding of the 90,000-$M_r$ protein to the affinity column (Figure 10C, lane 3), which indicated that the 90,000-$M_r$ protein recognized by mAb ME 20.4 represents the nuclear receptor for NGF.[212] We suggest that the 90,000-$M_r$ chromatin receptor in SKBr 5 cells corresponds to the 90,000-$M_r$ protein band that dissociated from the 230,000-$M_r$ receptor in the presence of NGF. In melanoma cells, which express the 230,000-$M_r$ receptor,

**TABLE 5**

**Analysis of the Amino Acids Present in the 230,000-$M_r$ Chromatin Receptor for NGF Compared to the Percentage of Amino Acids Present in the 75,000-$M_r$ Glycosylated Form of the Cell Surface Receptor**

| Amino acid | Chromatin receptor | | | Cell surface NGF receptor % of molecule[a] |
| | Picomoles | Residues in one 230,000-$M_r$ molecule | % of molecule | |
|---|---|---|---|---|
| ASX | 504 | 208 | 10.3 | 6.9 |
| GLX | 576 | 238 | 11.7 | 12.6 |
| SER | 110 | 46 | 2.2 | 8.4 |
| GLY | 310 | 128 | 6.3 | 8.2 |
| HIS | 274 | 113 | 5.6 | 1.9 |
| ARG | 250 | 103 | 5.1 | 4.4 |
| THR | 195 | 81 | 4.0 | 7.7 |
| ALA | 453 | 187 | 9.2 | 9.8 |
| PRO | 266 | 110 | 5.4 | 6.8 |
| TYR | 145 | 60 | 3.0 | 2.1 |
| VAL | 344 | 142 | 7.0 | 7.2 |
| MET | 68 | 28 | 1.4 | 0.9 |
| ILE | 183 | 75 | 3.7 | 2.1 |
| LEU | 529 | 219 | 10.8 | 8.4 |
| PHE | 219 | 90 | 4.5 | 0.9 |
| LYS | 483 | 200 | 9.8 | 2.6 |
| TRP | n.d.[b] | — | — | 1.1 |
| CYS | —[c] | —[c] | —[c] | 6.8 |

[a]  Amino acid composition was calculated according to the amino acid sequences predicted by Johnson et al. (1986) based on cDNA sequential analysis. The predicted molecular weight is 49,689.

[b]  *n.d.*, not determined.

[c]  Cysteine/cystine content was estimated by comparing cystine recovery of standards after acid hydrolysis and correcting cysteine for partial destruction during hydrolysis. Since hydrolysis losses are variable, only an approximate estimate of about 0.6 mol % or less was determined.

chromatin binding of NGF is several times lower than in SKBr 5 cells, which express predominantly the 90,000-$M_r$ chromatin receptor. We suggest that the 90,000-$M_r$ protein represents the NGF-binding subunit of the chromatin receptor.

### d. 35,000-$M_r$ Chromatin Receptor

Colorectal carcinoma cell line SW707 was found to express the high molecular weight cell surface receptor ($M_r$ 150,000), which is likely either to represent the product of the trk oncogene or a high molecular weight form of the low-affinity receptor. In addition to the 150,000-$M_r$ protein, a 45,000-$M_r$ protein was also immunoprecipitated from SW707 cells[176] (Figure 11, lanes 2 to 4). Whether the 45,000-$M_r$ protein represents a low molecular weight receptor for NGF or the degradation product of the high molecular weight receptor was not established. A low molecular weight protein ($M_r$ 35,000) was immunoprecipitated from the chromatin of SW707 cells[171] (Figure 11, lanes 1 and 3). Neither 230,000-$M_r$ protein nor 90,000-$M_r$ protein bands were immunoprecipitated from these cells. Since SW707 cell chromatin binds NGF, and the cells respond to NGF both at the transcriptional and replication levels (see sections F and G), we suggest that the 35,000-$M_r$ protein must be somehow involved in mediating NGF action on the nuclear level. Whether the 35,000-$M_r$ protein represents a subunit or a degradation product of a larger receptor remains to be established.

### e. Scatchard Analysis of NGF Binding to Particular Species of Chromatin Receptor

Identification of specific proteins by immunoprecipitation of chromatin isolated from different cell lines with mAb 20.4 developed against the cell surface NGF receptor suggests that NGF taken up by the nucleus may interact with this receptor protein(s). This suggestion is strongly supported by the fact that after "saturation" of the chromatin with NGF, mAb ME 20.4 did not recognize the receptor (Figure 10C). Alternatively, "saturation" of the chromatin with mAb ME 20.4 inhibits binding of NGF. Scatchard analysis of the kinetics of NGF binding to the chromatin of HS 294, SW707 (Figure 12),[175] and SKBr 5 cells (not shown) indicated saturable chromatin binding of NGF at NGF concentrations of 40 p$M$ to 4 n$M$. The dissociation constant ($K_D$) for HS 294 melanoma cell chromatin receptor (230,000 $M_r$) calculated based on the linear plot was 241 p$M$, with $1.6 \times 10^9$ binding sites per microgram DNA. In SW707 cells, two classes of NGF binding sites were distinguished, one with $K_D = 333$ p$M$ ($7.1 \times 10^8$/µg DNA) and another with $K_D = 1718$ p$M$ ($1.6 \times 10^9$). In SKBr 5 cells, one class of NGF binding sites was detected with $K_D = 150$ p$M$ ($2 \times 10^9$ binding sites per microgram DNA). In control experiments chromatin isolated from SW948 colorectal carcinoma cell line, which does not express the NGF chromatin receptors, did not bind NGF specifically (not shown).

### 2. EGF Receptors

mAb 425 against the EGF receptor immunoprecipitated the 170,000-$M_r$ cell surface receptor (not shown) and the 250,000-$M_r$ protein from the chromatin of the colorectal carcinoma cell line SW948[220] (Figure 13, lanes 1, 3, 5, 7). The 250,000-$M_r$ chromatin protein did not crossreact with mAb 20.4 against NGF receptor (Figure 13, lane 6), nor with nonspecific antibody P3×63Ag8 (Figure 13, lanes 2 and 4). Since mAb 425 blocks binding of $^{125}$I-EGF to the chromatin, it is likely that the 250,000-$M_r$ chromatin protein represents the EGF chromatin receptor.

### 3. Insulin Receptors

The insulin receptor is present on the surface of almost all normal and tumor cells. It is composed of α (135,000 $M_r$) and β (95,000 $M_r$) subunits.

Nuclear uptake and chromatin binding of $^{125}$I-insulin (Table 1D) suggested that a chromatin receptor may be expressed in the nucleus. In order to identify the

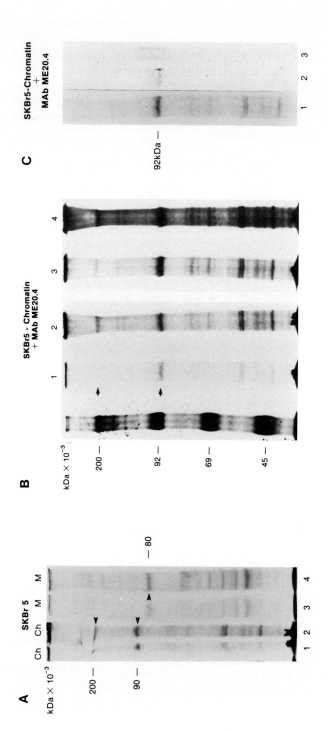

**FIGURE 10.** SDS-PAGE (7.5 polyacrylamide gel) and autoradiographic detection of chromatin proteins immunoprecipitated by mAb ME 20.4 from [$^{35}$S]methionine-labeled SKBr5 breast carcinoma chromatin. (A) SDS-polyacrylamide gel electrophoresis (7.5 polyacrylamide gel) and autoradiographic detection of proteins immunoprecipitated by mAb ME 20.4 from [$^{35}$S]methionine-labeled SKBr5 breast carcinoma cell membranes (M) and chromatin (Ch). Lanes 1 and 3 represent material obtained from cells not exposed to NGF, and lanes 2 and 4 from cells exposed to NGF (24 h, 10 ng/ml). (B) Chromatin was isolated from cells not exposed (lanes 1 and 3) or exposed to NGF (10 ng/ml) (lanes 2 and 4). Lanes 1, 2 and 3, 4 represent 24 h and 48 h, respectively, of autoradiogram exposure. (C) *Eco*RI-digested chromatin was immunoprecipitated with mAb ME 20.4 prior to (lane 1) or after (lane 2) affinity chromatography on mAb ME 20.4-protein A-agarose column. Pre-exposure of the isolated chromatin to NGF (20 ng/ml) abolished binding of the receptor to the mAb ME 20.4 affinity column (lane 3). (From Rakowicz-Szulczynska, E. M., *J. Cell. Physiol.*, 154, 71, 1992. With permission.)

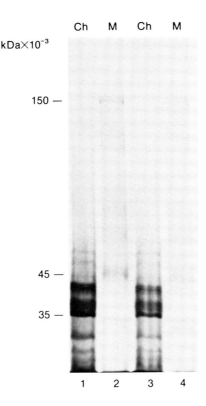

**FIGURE 11.** SDS-PAGE (10% polyacrylamide gel) of [$^{35}$S]methionine-labeled chromatin (Ch) or membrane (M) proteins immunoprecipitated from SW707 colorectal carcinoma cells by mAb ME 20.4. Material was obtained from $15 \times 10^6$ cells (lanes 1 and 2) or $10 \times 10^6$ cells (lanes 3 and 4).

chromatin receptor, a technique different than that used to identify the NGF and EGF receptor was applied. Chromatin proteins from SW948, SW707 colorectal carcinoma, and WM266-4 melanoma cells were electrophoretically separated and electroblotted onto the nitrocellulose filters. Filters were incubated with $^{125}$I-insulin, which revealed 45,000-$M_r$ chromatin protein specifically bound to $^{125}$I-insulin (Figure 14). We suggest that the 45,000-$M_r$ protein represents the chromatin receptor for insulin.

## E. MECHANISM OF NUCLEAR TRANSLOCATION OF GROWTH FACTORS: STUDIES IN A CELL-FREE SYSTEM

### 1. Nuclear Translocation of Growth Factors

The rational mechanism of the nuclear translocation of growth factors might involve covalent attachment of the growth factor to the cell surface receptor, followed by endocytosis and nuclear uptake of the whole complex. Such a possibility is, however, eliminated by the fact that all tested growth factors, when extracted from the chromatin, exhibited the same electrophoretic mobility as free growth factors. The results eliminate a possibility that the tested growth factors are taken

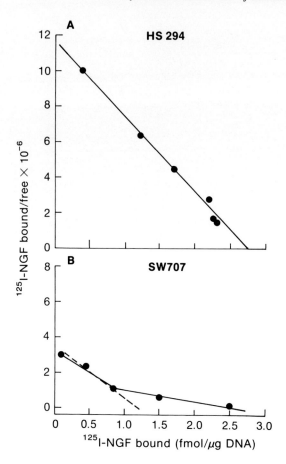

**FIGURE 12.** Scatchard plot of $^{125}$I-NGF binding to the isolated chromatin from HS294 (A) and SW707 (B) cells. The chromatin equivalent of 1 μg DNA was adsorbed to the wells of the microliter plates and incubated for 1 h at room temperature with various concentrations of NGF (40 p*M* to 4 n*M*). Data are means of triplicate determinations of binding, with nonspecific binding subtracted. The data were plotted according to Scatchard. (From Rakowicz-Szulczynska, E. M., Herlyn, M., and Koprowski, H., *Cancer Res.*, 48, 7200, 1988. With permission of American Association for Cancer Research, Inc.)

up by the nucleus as covalently bound to the cell surface receptor. In addition, even in cells exposed to NGF, the cell surface receptor was never found in the cell nucleus. The possibility of nuclear translocation of the cell surface receptor may be completely eliminated in the case of NGF receptors, based on comparative analysis of amino acid composition (Table 5). Whether the EGF or insulin chromatin receptors do not originate from the cell surface was not determined. We suggest, therefore, that at least NGF penetrates the nucleus of the target cell, as the free protein unchanged or activated in the cytoplasm.

To test whether free growth factors are able to penetrate the cell nucleus, or if the plasma membrane receptor or another cytoplasmic protein(s) are needed as vehicles for the nuclear translocation of growth factors, experiments were performed

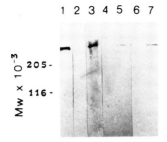

**FIGURE 13.** SDS-PAGE (7% polyacrylamide gel) of [$^{35}$S]methionine-labeled protein immunoprecipitated from SW948 colorectal carcinoma cells with mAb 425 (lanes 1, 3, 5, and 7), anti-NGF receptor mAb 20.4 (lane 6), and control antibody P3 × 63Ag8 (lanes 2 and 4). Lanes 6 and 7 show the results of immunoprecipitation with mAb 20.4 (lane 6) followed by immunoprecipitation with mAb 425 (lane 7). Lanes 1 to 3 were Coomassie blue stained, and lanes 4 to 7 were autoradiographed. Results are from four independent experiments. The immunoprecipitated protein (chromatin receptor for EGF) exhibits an $M_r$ of 250,000. (From Rakowicz-Szulczynska, E. M., Otwiaska, D. Rodeck, U., and Koprowski, H., *Arch. Biochem. Biophys.*, 268, 456, 1989. With permission.)

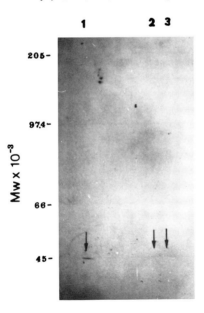

**FIGURE 14.** Insulin-binding chromatin proteins from SW948 (lane 1), WM266-4 (lane 2), and SW707 cells (lane 3) separated by SDS-PAGE and blotted onto nitrocellulose.

in a cell-free system.[173] Four variants of experiments were performed with each of the tested growth factors.

1. Nuclei were isolated from tumor cells that accumulate the given growth factor and incubated with $^{125}$I-growth factor in a synthetic medium containing: 250 m$M$ sucrose, 20 m$M$ Tris-HCl (pH 7.8), 10 m$M$ MgCl$_2$, 0.5% BSA.

2.    Synthetic medium was replaced by pure, membrane-free cytosol, prepared in
      the same synthetic medium as in experiment 1.
3.    Synthetic medium was replaced by crude membrane-containing cytoplasm.
4.    Synthetic medium contained the microsomal (membrane) fraction.

$^{125}$I-NGF and $^{125}$I-PDGF were taken up by isolated nuclei in all four variants
of experiments. Nuclear uptake was highest in the synthetic medium and is referred
to as 100% uptake (Table 4).

When incubation with $^{125}$I-NGF[173] or $^{125}$I-PDGF was performed in the presence
of the membrane-free cytosol, or in the crude, membrane-containing cytoplasm,
nuclear translocation of both growth factors was inhibited by more than 50%.
Microsomal fraction, when added to the synthetic medium, inhibited nuclear translocation of both growth factors to a lesser degree than the crude cytoplasm or pure
cytosol (Table 6).

The results obtained indicate that free $^{125}$I-NGF and $^{125}$I-PDGF probably, in a
native form, penetrate the cell nucleus. Moreover, it seems that the cell surface
receptor which is present in the cytoplasm (or microsomal fraction) may competitively inhibit nuclear translocation of both growth factors. Since microsomal fraction inhibited nuclear translocation in a lower degree than the membrane-free cytosol, we suspected that an additional component other than the membrane-bound
receptor competitively inhibited nuclear translocation of $^{125}$I-NGF and $^{125}$I-PDGF.
When the cytosol from the target cells (the cells that express appropriate receptor)
was replaced by the cytosol from non-target cells (the cells that do not express the
receptor), inhibition of nuclear uptake of NGF was not observed.

$^{125}$I-EGF[172] or $^{125}$I-insulin,[172,235] in contrast to $^{125}$I-NGF and $^{125}$I-PDGF, did not
penetrate the nucleus in the presence of the synthetic medium or the membrane-
free cytosol (Table 6). However, when the nuclei were incubated with $^{125}$I-EGF or
$^{125}$I-insulin in the presence of crude cytoplasm, or microsomal fraction-containing
synthetic medium, both EGF and insulin were efficiently translocated to the cell
nucleus (Table 6). The results suggest that EGF and insulin either are activated by
binding to the membrane receptor or undergo cytoplasmic modifications prior to
the nuclear translocation.

To determine whether chromatin-bound $^{125}$I-growth factors had undergone any
degradation, chromatin proteins isolated from nuclei incubated at room temperature
for 2 h with $^{125}$I-growth factor in crude cytoplasm, pure cytosol, or synthetic medium
were subjected to electrophoresis. Figure 15 represents an example of growth factor-
degradation analysis, using NGF as a model. The chromatin-bound $^{125}$I-NGF showed
the same electrophoretic mobility as free NGF, suggesting that NGF is taken up by
the nucleus and bound to the chromatin in nondegraded form.[173]

Nonspecific adsorption of $^{125}$I-NGF or $^{125}$I-PDGF to the nuclear membrane,
nonspecific diffusion of these growth factors through the nuclear membrane, or
nonspecific translocation through the nuclear membrane resulting from damage
during isolation of nuclei, may be eliminated, since $^{125}$I-EGF of a molecular weight
($M_r$ 7,000) much lower than NGF ($M_r$ 26,000) or PDGF ($M_r$ 30,000), was not
translocated to the nucleus in a synthetic medium. In addition to the tested growth
factors, nuclear uptake of a high molecular weight protein (BSA, 66,000) was tested

## TABLE 6
## Nuclear Translocation of Different Growth Factors
## in a Cell-Free System

| Nuclei origin | Growth factor | Experiment | [125]I-growth factor molecules per nucleus[a] | | |
| | | | Nuclear membrane | Nucleoplasm | Chromatin |
|---|---|---|---|---|---|
| *Colorectal Carcinoma* | | | | | |
| SW948 | EGF | A | 100 | 50 | 5 |
| | | B | 100 | 60 | 10 |
| | | C | 400 | 250 | 2,500 |
| | | D | 300 | 150 | 1,400 |
| *Colorectal Carcinoma* | | | | | |
| SW948 | Insulin | A | 100 | 180 | 330 |
| | | B | 95 | 150 | 350 |
| | | C | 250 | 140 | 40,000 |
| | | D | 260 | 125 | 37,000 |
| *Melanoma* | | | | | |
| HS294 | NGF | A | 400 | 580 | 33,800 |
| | | B | 150 | 180 | 14,800 |
| | | C | 125 | 200 | 14,000 |
| | | D | 100 | 200 | 28,000 |
| *Melanoma* | | | | | |
| WM266-4 | PDGF | A | 80 | 50 | 2,500 |
| | | B | 40 | 40 | 1,200 |
| | | C | 50 | 60 | 1,100 |
| | | D | 70 | 50 | 1,950 |

[a]  Nuclei were incubated 1 h at 20°C, with [125]I-growth factor (10 ng/ml), in the synthetic medium (A), membrane-free cytosol (B), crude, membrane-containing cytoplasm (C), or synthetic medium plus microsomal fraction (D). Mean from three experiments; SD = 10 to 15%.

in control experiments. [125]I-BSA in a tenfold excess mixed with [125]I-NGF, and tested simultaneously in each experiment, was not taken up by the nucleus in any of the experiments, which further confirms specificity of NGF and PDGF translocation across the nuclear membrane.

## 2. Analyses of the Cytoplasmic Component Involved in Inhibition of NGF Nuclear Translocation

Inhibition of [125]I-NGF nuclear uptake by the membrane-free cytosol from cells expressing the NGF receptor (Table 6), but not by the cytosol from cells negative for receptor expression (not shown), suggested the involvement of an NGF receptor in this inhibition. To test this hypothesis, we mixed cytosol derived from A875 cells with mAb ME 20.4, which competitively inhibits binding of NGF to its receptor,[210] and tested the mixture for its effect on [125]I-NGF nuclear uptake. In the presence of mAb 20.4, nuclear uptake of [125]I-NGF was only slightly inhibited, compared with the strong inhibition by cytosol alone (not shown). Thus, the NGF

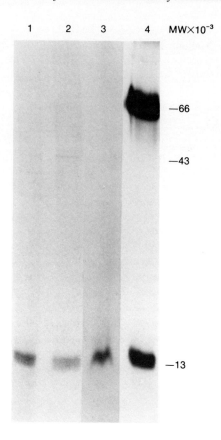

**FIGURE 15.** Autoradiogram of SDS-PAGE (15% polyacrylamide gel) of $^{125}$I-NGF incorporated into the chromatin of A875 melanoma cell nuclei incubated (2 h at room temperature) with $^{125}$I-NGF (10 ng/ml) and $^{125}$I-BSA (50 ng/ml) in membrane-free cytosol (lane 1), crude cytoplasm (lane 2), and chemically defined medium (lane 3). Lane 4 shows a mixture of free $^{125}$I-NGF and $^{125}$I-BSA ($^{125}$I-BSA can be seen at the top). Only $^{125}$I-NGF specifically enters the nuclei. (From Rakowicz-Szulczynska, E. M., Linnenbach, A., and Koprowski, H., *Mol. Carcinogen.*, 2, 47, 1989. With permission.)

receptor present in the membrane-free cytosol interacts with $^{125}$I-NGF, inhibiting uptake of $^{125}$I-NGF by isolated nuclei. Since mAb 20.4 binds to the cytosolic receptor, it promotes nuclear uptake of $^{125}$I-NGF.

In further analyses of NGF-binding cytosolic components, $^{125}$I-NGF was incubated with cytosol of unlabeled cells, which resulted in the formation of a $^{125}$I-NGF-containing precipitate.[173,249] In a control experiment, $^{125}$I-NGF was mixed with membrane-containing cytoplasm. The precipitate formed was removed by centrifugation together with the membrane (microsomal) fraction and tested by electron microscopy (Figure 16B). Comparison of the two micrographs indicates that the precipitate formed by NGF in membrane-free cytosol was homogeneous and contained no microsomal (membrane) contaminants seen after precipitation of the membrane-containing cytoplasm (see Figure 16A). To test the composition of

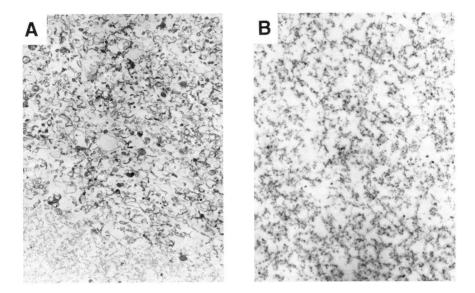

**FIGURE 16.** Electron microscopy of the membrane-containing fraction precipitated by NGF from the crude cytoplasm of A875 melanoma cells before incubation with NGF (A) and of the precipitate obtained from the membrane-free cytosol incubated with NGF (B). (Original magnification × 66,000.)

the precipitate for the presence of RNA, unlabeled NGF was incubated with cytosol of cells labeled with [³H]uridine. Approximately 3% of the cytoplasmic [³H]uridine was precipitated by NGF, suggesting that the precipitate contained RNA. Using a [³²P]CTP-labeled NGF receptor cDNA probe, Northern blot analysis of RNA extracted from the NGF precipitate revealed an intact 3.5-kb species (Figure 17, lanes 1 and 2) characteristic of NGF receptor mRNA[173] (Figure 17, lane 3). In a control experiment, a [³²P]CTP-labeled cDNA probe for α-enolase, which is constitutively expressed at high levels, did not hybridize with the RNA of the NGF precipitate on the same filter (Figure 17, lane 4), but hybridized with the control RNA (Figure 17, lane 5). The results indicate that NGF precipitates mRNA for its receptor with a very high specificity.[249]

The precipitate formed by NGF in the cytoplasm of A875 melanoma cells labeled with [³⁵S]methionine and [³⁵S]cysteine contained both amino acids, suggesting that proteins are also precipitated by NGF. The precipitate was analyzed electrophoretically by SDS-PAGE under reducing conditions, which revealed a 78-kDa protein band (Figure 18B, lane 1). When the precipitate was formed by ¹²⁵I-NGF in the unlabeled cytosol, two bands migrating at 78 kDa (major band) and at 240 kDa (minor band) (Figure 18B, lane 2) were detected electrophoretically. Since the NGF monomer is 13 kDa, we concluded that these complexes resisted dissociation by SDS and 2-mercaptoethanol. Thus, the 78-kDa band might represent a monomer of NGF bound to the synthesized 65-kDa surface receptor, and the 240-kDa species may contain the 13-kDa NGF monomer bound to the 230-kDa chromatin

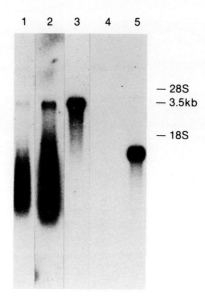

**FIGURE 17.** Northern blot hybridization of RNA precipitated by NGF from A875 melanoma cell cytoplasm (lanes 1, 2, and 4) and of control RNA from NGF receptor-expressing cells (WM135 melanoma) (lanes 3 and 5). All filters were hybridized with the $^{32}$P-labeled cDNA probe for the NGF receptor gene. Lanes 1 and 2 represent 12-h and 48-h exposure. The same filter (lanes 2 and 3) was dehybridized and rehybridized to the α-enolase cDNA probe (lanes 4 and 5). RNA precipitated by NGF represents mRNA for NGF receptor (lanes 1 and 2), which does not have impurities of the abundant mRNA of α-enolase (Figure 4). Control RNA from WM135 cells hybridizes with both cDNA probe for NGF receptor (lane 3) and cDNA probe for a-enolase (lane 5). (From Rakowicz-Szulczynska, E. M., Linnenbach, A., and Koprowski, H., *Mol. Carcinogen.*, 2, 47, copyright © 1989. With permission of Wiley-Liss, division of John Wiley and Sons, Inc.)

receptor.[173] In the control experiment (Figure 18A), cytosol was prepared from [$^{35}$S]methionine, [$^{35}$S]cystein-labeled colorectal carcinoma SW707 cells, which express 150,000-$M_r$ cell surface receptor. NGF precipitated a band of the $M_r$ 170,000 to 180,000 (probably receptor-NGF complex) which confirms the specificity of the precipitation procedure. After the precipitates were removed from the SW707 (Figure 18A, lane 1), or from A875 (Figure 18B, lanes 1 and 2) cell cytosol, no precipitate was further formed by NGF (Figure 18A, lane 2; Figure 18B, lane 3).

To analyze whether NGF binds selectively to the receptor (or receptors) or also to other cytoplasmic proteins, in some experiments the cross-linking agent dimethyl suberimidate was added after the pure cytosol was mixed with $^{125}$I-NGF. The precipitate formed with A875 cell cytosol contained a $^{125}$I-NGF bound to a 78-kDa complex (Figure 18C), which appeared to represent the monomeric complex also observed in the absence of cross-linking agent (Figure 18B) and a 175-kDa species, which may represent a dimeric form of the cell surface NGF receptor bound to dimeric NGF (26 kDa) (Figure 18C). The cross-linked form of the high molecular weight chromatin receptor appears as the unseparated band at the top of the gel.[173]

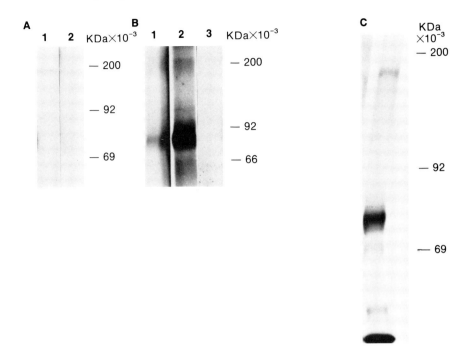

**FIGURE 18.** (A) Autoradiogram of SDS-PAGE (10% polyacrylamide gel) under reducing conditions of the precipitate formed after incubation of unlabeled NGF (2 μg/cytosol from 20 × 10⁶ cells) with [³⁵S]methionine- and [³⁵S]cysteine-labeled membrane-free cytosol from SW707 colorectal carcinoma cells (lane 1); no protein was precipitated by NGF from the cytosol from which the precipitate (lane 1) was removed. (B) Analysis of the precipitate formed by NGF in the [³⁵S]methionine, [³⁵S]cysteine-labeled cytosol (lane 1), or by ¹²⁵I-NGF in the unlabeled cytosol (lane 2) from A875 melanoma cells. No protein was precipitated by ¹²⁵I-NGF from the cytosol (lane 3) after removal of the precipitate (lane 2). (C) Autoradiogram of SDS-PAGE (7.5% polyacrylamide gel) of the precipitate formed after incubation of ¹²⁵I-NGF with membrane-free cytoplasm in the presence of cross-linking agent (dimethyl suberimidate). (From Rakowicz-Szulczynska, E. M., Linnenbach, A., and Koprowski, H., *Mol. Carcinogen.*, 2, 47, copyright © 1989. With permission of Wiley-Liss, division of John Wiley and Sons, Inc.)

To determine whether the NGF-containing cytosolic fraction remaining after centrifugation of the NGF-precipitate also contained NGF-binding proteins, the fraction was chromatographed on a Sepharose (CL4B) protein A-anti-NGF IgG column. The eluted fraction contained a ³⁵S-labeled 42-kDa protein that migrated as a single band in SDS-PAGE. Chromatography of the cytosol on a Sepharose (CL4B)-protein A-anti-actin IgG column identified that protein as actin. A possibility of NGF interaction with actin has also been considered by other authors.[207]

The results obtained indicated that the receptor which is being synthesized in the cytoplasm is able to bind NGF in a cell-free system. Binding of ¹²⁵I-NGF to the molecules of the synthesized receptor results in the precipitation of the complex containing both the synthesized receptor and the corresponding mRNA. The reaction of precipitation is very specific and allowed the development of new methods for the detection and isolation of the synthesized receptor for the growth factor and mRNA encoding of this receptor in a one-step procedure.[249]

## 3. Analysis of NGF Binding to the Synthesizing NGF Receptor in Intact Cells

To test whether interaction of the growth factor with the synthesizing receptor at the polysomal level represents an artifact occurring only in a cell-free system, or instead represents a phenomenon occurring in intact cells, cytoplasm was isolated from cells incubated for 2 h with unlabeled NGF and tested for the ability to inhibit the nuclear uptake of $^{125}$I-NGF.[173] No inhibition of nuclear transport of $^{125}$I-NGF was observed, in contrast with the inhibition observed by cytoplasm isolated from cells not preincubated with NGF. These experiments suggest that NGF taken up by cells binds to intracellular (synthesized on polysomes) receptors that can no longer bind the exogenously added $^{125}$I-NGF.

Nuclear uptake of $^{125}$I-NGF in cells preincubated with NGF for 1 h or 3 h was higher than that in cells not previously exposed to NGF (Table 7), which may suggest that the NGF receptor which was actively synthesized on polysomes after saturation with NGF did not bind $^{125}$I-NGF. To test this possibility further, nuclear uptake of $^{125}$I-NGF was tested in intact A875 cells incubated for 1 h with cyclo-heximide (which inhibits protein synthesis at the translocation or transpeptidation level) or puromycin (which prematurely releases mRNAs from ribosomes) or actinomycin D (which inhibits transcription of rRNA and mRNA), and cells were then exposed to $^{125}$I-NGF for 1 h. The results in Table 7 indicate that nuclear uptake and chromatin binding of $^{125}$I-NGF increased after 1 h exposure to each inhibitor as compared with uptake observed in cells incubated in culture medium alone. The highest increase in chromatin accumulation of $^{125}$I-NGF was observed using actinomycin D. Since the total number of internalized molecules did not change after 1 h of exposure to inhibitors of protein biosynthesis, an increase in nuclear accumulation must be done for more effective translocation of $^{125}$I-NGF from the cytoplasm to the nucleus. It is likely that actively synthesized NGF receptor binds the NGF taken up by the cell and competitively inhibits the nuclear uptake. When the synthesis of this receptor is inhibited, nuclear translocation of NGF is not restricted and more $^{125}$I-NGF binds to the chromatin.

To establish whether intracellular NGF uptake results in an irreversible internalization of the surface NGF receptor, its degradation, or nuclear translocation, cells were preincubated simultaneously with unlabeled NGF (to induce receptor internalization) and with cycloheximide (to inhibit *de novo* receptor synthesis). With a 1 h preincubation, the amount of $^{125}$I-NGF taken up by intact cells did not change compared with cells incubated without cycloheximide and NGF, and the amount of $^{125}$I-NGF bound to the chromatin increased (Table 5). These experiments suggested that NGF cell surface receptors are internalized together with NGF, but are next recycled to the cell surface and are still able to bind new molecules of $^{125}$I-NGF. To eliminate the possibility that $^{125}$I-NGF was internalized independently of the expression of the cell surface receptor, cells were exposed to inhibitors of

**TABLE 7**

**Chromatin Binding of $^{125}$I-NGF in Intact A875 Melanoma Cells After Preincubation with Unlabeled NGF or Inhibitors of Protein Biosynthesis Followed by 1-h Exposure to $^{125}$I-NGF**

| Preincubation | Internalized molecules/cell | | Chromatin-bound molecules/cell[a] | |
|---|---|---|---|---|
| | *Time at preincubation* | | | |
| | 1 h | 3 h | 1 h | 3 h |
| Culture medium | 5,500 ± 250 | 8,900 ± 270 | 480 ± 20 | 1,000 |
| NGF (50 ng/ml) | 5,200 ± 150 | 9,000 ± 250 | 750 ± 50 | 1,700 |
| Cycloheximide (50 μg/ml) | 5,400 ± 200 | 500 ± 50 | 480 ± 30 | 100 ± 10 |
| Puromycin (200 μg/ml) | 5,000 ± 100 | 520 ± 50 | 750 ± 25 | 90 ± 10 |
| Actinomycin D (20 μg/ml) | 5,450 ± 150 | 450 ± 20 | 1,000 ± 50 | 80 ± 10 |
| NGF (50 ng/ml) + cycloheximide (50 μg/ml) | 5,500 ± 100 | 520 ± 50 | 800 ± 50 | 150 ± 30 |

[a]  The mean ± SE of five experiments.

protein biosynthesis for 3 h and then incubated with $^{125}$I-NGF. This long preincubation resulted in a decreased number of internalized molecules to 10% (Table 5). Thus, the internalized NGF receptor recycles to the cell surface with a half-life of less than 3 h.

In the events that follow entry of NGF into the intact cell, a fraction of the growth factor is bound by the intracytoplasmic receptor being synthesized on the polysome. Another fraction of NGF is taken up from the cytoplasm and is transported to the nucleus, where it is bound to chromatin. We suspect that binding of NGF to the synthesized receptor may result in intracellular precipitation of the polysomal complexes involved in receptor synthesis, which consequently may inhibit expression of the receptor on the cell surface. This internal loop may potentially downregulate the receptor when the cell is exposed to a high concentration of the growth factors. Alternatively, binding of NGF to the synthesized receptor may stabilize mRNA. The following experiments support the latest hypothesis: A875 melanoma cells were exposed for 3 h to actinomycin D alone, or actinomycin D plus unlabeled NGF (10 ng/ml) followed by 1 h incubation with $^{125}$I-NGF (Table 8). Cells preincubated with actinomycin D incorporated only 7% of the amount of $^{125}$I-NGF internalized by control cells exposed to neither actinomycin D nor NGF. Cells incubated with actinomycin D plus NGF internalized 56% of $^{125}$I-NGF internalized by control cells. The experiments indicate that NGF stabilized expression of its receptor. We suggest that the mechanism of stabilization involved interaction of NGF at the translational (polysomal) level.

TABLE 8
Internalization of [125]I-NGF During 1-h
Incubation of A875 Melanoma Cells not
Preincubated and Preincubated for 3 h with
Actinomycin D (10 µg/ml) or
Actinomycin D and NGF (10 ng/ml)

| Preincubation | [125]I-NGF (cpm/10⁶ cells)[a] | Percentage (%) |
|---|---|---|
| — | 20,520 | 100 |
| Actinomycin | 1,460 | 7 |
| Actinomycin D + NGF | 11,400 | 56 |

[a]   Total amount incorporated into cytoplasm, nucleoplasm,
      nuclear membranes, and chromatin; data are given as mean
      from two experiments; SD = 5%.

The interaction of NGF with the synthesizing receptor and nuclear uptake of nondegraded NGF are difficult to explain at the level of cell compartmentation. NGF is probably taken up by cells through receptor-mediated endocytosis. From the endosomes, the receptor may be released and recycled to the cell surface. At least a fraction of NGF is released from the membrane system and translocated in nondegraded form to the nucleus. The mechanism of this translocation requires further study. The interaction between the synthesizing receptor, which like all secreted proteins must contain a signal peptide in order to be transported into the lumen of the endoplasmic reticulum, and NGF also remains unclear. However, this interaction occurs efficiently in a cell-free system after centrifugation of membranes. Electron microscopy showed that the precipitate is 100% homogeneous and free of membrane contamination (Figure 16B). Even under hypotonic condition, it seems unlikely that synthesizing receptor is released without a vesicle coating pinched off from the endoplasmic reticulum. We cannot exclude the possibility that NGF interacts with two types of cell surface receptors, one present on the cell surface (translocated during synthesis into the lumen) and another present in cytoplasm (synthesized on free polysomes). The hypothetical cytoplasmic receptor might play an additional role in the growth regulation of cells.

## F. EFFECT OF GROWTH FACTORS TRANSLOCATED TO THE NUCLEUS ON RNA AND DNA SYNTHESIS

### 1. RNA Synthesis in Intact Cells

Cells that express appropriate cell surface and the nuclear receptors were exposed for 1 h or 24 h to each of the tested growth factors (NGF, PDGF, EGF, or insulin) in the presence of [³H]uridine (Figure 19A). Cells were next solubilized in 10 m$M$ Tris-HCl and the amounts of [³H]uridine incorporated into the TCA-precipitable cytoplasmic fraction, nucleoplasm, and chromatin were estimated and used as an exponent of RNA synthesis. Exposure of SW707 colorectal carcinoma cells (Figure 19A) or any other cell line with appropriate receptors (not shown) to EGF or insulin resulted in slightly increased RNA synthesis (by 2%) compared to cells not exposed to any of the growth factors. Whether the slightly increased RNA synthesis after cell exposure to EGF or insulin reflects an effect of the growth factors on transcription of specific genes remains to be established.

In contrast to EGF and insulin, NGF tested in A875 melanoma cells which express the 230,000-$M_r$ chromatin receptor and PDGF (in melanoma WM266-4) exerted very strong but opposite effects on RNA synthesis: NGF inhibited RNA synthesis, and PDGF activated it. Even in the presence of a low concentration of NGF (0.5 ng/ml), RNA synthesis was 27% lower than in cells not exposed to NGF. NGF at the concentration of 1 ng/ml decreased RNA synthesis by 48%, and at the concentration of 5 to 10 ng/ml by 50%. Higher concentrations of NGF (20 to 100 ng/ml) did not inhibit RNA synthesis by more than 50%.

PDGF at the concentration of 5 ng/ml activated RNA synthesis by 100%, and at the concentration of 10 ng/ml by 200% (Figure 19A). Higher concentration of PDGF (20 to 100 ng/ml) activated RNA synthesis by an additional 30 to 50%.

Since experiments with intact cells do not allow for distinguishing which of two receptors (the cell surface or the nuclear) expressed by cells is involved in mediating growth factor action on RNA-synthesis level, the next experiments were performed in a cell-free system, using isolated nuclei.

## 2. RNA Synthesis in a Cell-Free System

Since EGF and insulin do not penetrate isolated nuclei (Table 3) and also do not affect significantly RNA synthesis in intact cells (Figure 19A), our studies were concentrated on NGF and PDGF.

Exposure of A875 melanoma cell nuclei that express the 230,000-$M_r$ receptor to NGF resulted in inhibition of RNA synthesis (Figure 19B), as determined by measuring [$^{32}$P]UTP incorporation into the chromatin-bound RNA. Effect of NGF was dependent on concentration, and at the NGF concentration 10 ng/ml, RNA synthesis was inhibited by 52%. Since even an inhibition of several unique genes would not affect RNA synthesis by more than 12 to 15%, we suspected that expression of rRNA, which represents the bulk of the synthesized RNA, must be affected by NGF. To check this hypothesis, the [$^{32}$P]UTP-labeled RNA synthesized by the nuclei incubated in the presence or absence of NGF was hybridized to the plasmid DNA containing the rDNA. The transcription level of rDNA was 70% lower in the nuclei exposed to NGF than in the nuclei not exposed (Figure 19B).

The control experiment was performed with the nuclei of SW948 colorectal carcinoma cells that do not express the nuclear receptor. NGF did not bind to the chromatin and did not modulate rRNA synthesis in these nuclei, which suggests that only the nuclear receptor for NGF mediates the inhibitory effect of NGF on rRNA synthesis.

In the experiments with PDGF, nuclei were isolated from WM266-4 melanoma cells that *in vitro* accumulate $^{125}$I-PDGF in the nucleus. Since the PDGF-binding chromatin protein (receptor) was never identified, we can only speculate that such

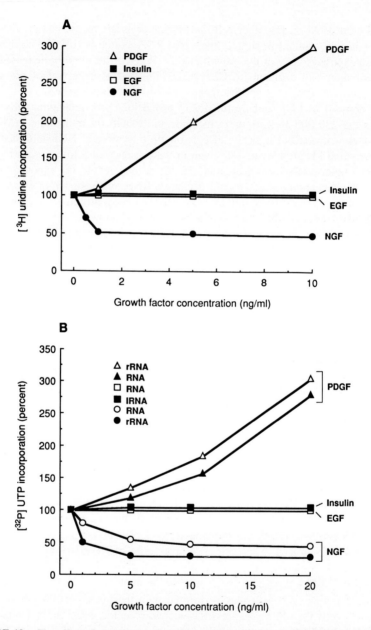

**FIGURE 19.** The effect of growth factors on RNA synthesis in intact cells (A) and in a cell-free system (B). In (A), A875 melanoma cells were exposed to NGF (10 ng/ml), WM266-4 melanoma cells were exposed to PDGF (10 ng/ml), and SW948 colorectal carcinoma cells were exposed to EGF or insulin (10 ng/ml). All cell lines express the cell surface and the chromatin receptor for the tested growth factors. In (A), incubation with [³H]uridine was performed for 24 h at 37°C. In (B), nuclei were isolated from the same lines and incubated with [³²P]UTP for 1 h at 20°C according to the above pattern. [³²P]UTP incorporated into TCA-insoluble fraction represents total RNA synthesis. A fraction of [³²P]UTP-RNA hybridizing to the probe for rDNA represents rRNA synthesis.

a protein exists. PDGF activated RNA synthesis by 180% and rRNA by 210% (Figure 19B). In control nuclei, isolated from SW948 cells that do not accumulate PDGF in the nucleus (do not express the PDGF receptor), PDGF did not exert any effect on rRNA synthesis. The stimulatory effect of PDGF on rRNA synthesis is similar to the effect of FGF described by Bouche et al. in Chapter 2.

The obtained results indicate that NGF and PDGF can directly affect rRNA synthesis. Both NGF and PDGF penetrate nuclei isolated from cells that in intact state accumulate or do not accumulate these growth factors in the chromatin. However, only in these nuclei that express chromatin receptor, do NGF and PDGF bind to the chromatin and exert effect on rRNA synthesis. It is likely that an expression of several unique genes may also be modulated by NGF and PDGF. Since particular unique genes are expressed in extremely low quantities, they do not affect total RNA-synthesis level. Instead, Northern blot analysis must be performed in the future, using a cDNA probe for specific genes.

## G. ANTAGONISTIC EFFECT OF NGF ON PDGF-ACTIVATED TRANSCRIPTION OF rDNA AND TUMOR CELL PROLIFERATION

Studies on the effect of one selected growth factor on RNA synthesis and on cell growth represent an *in vitro* model which does not resemble the situation *in vivo,* when growth of neoplastic cells and maintenance of their neoplastic state is regulated by several endogenous and exogenous growth factors. However, as long as we do not know which unique genes are regulated directly after binding of growth factors to the chromatin of the target cells and which are activated indirectly by second messengers, we also cannot predict the total effect exerted by all growth factors, for which the specific receptors are expressed on the target cells. However, since one of the genes (rDNA) is known to be directly regulated by NGF and PDGF (and fibroblast growth factor; see Chapter 2), we established a model system which allowed us to analyze the cell response to each of these two growth factors alone and to both growth factors together.[172] Colorectal carcinoma SW707 cells that express both receptors (for NGF and PDGF) on the cell surface and accumulate both growth factors in the cell nucleus were used in these studies.

Analysis of RNA synthesis in intact SW707 cells indicated that RNA synthesis is activated by PDGF (by approximately 200%) but inhibited by NGF by 55% (Figure 20A). When PDGF and NGF were added simultaneously to the cell culture, RNA synthesis was inhibited by 50%; i.e., to similar levels as in the presence of NGF alone (Figure 20A). A similar effect of both growth factors was observed in a cell free system, when the nuclei isolated from SW707 cells, which express the $35,000\text{-}M_r$ chromatin receptor for NGF, were exposed to NGF or PDGF alone and to both growth factors simultaneously: NGF inhibited incorporation of [$^{32}$P]UTP into RNA; PDGF activated it; and, in the presence of PDGF plus NGF, incorporation of [$^{32}$P]UTP into RNA was similar to that in the presence of NGF alone (Figure 20B). Hybridization of the [$^{32}$P]UTP-labeled RNA synthesized in the presence or absence of these growth factors to the probe of rDNA confirmed that NGF antagonized the activatory effect of PDGF on rRNA synthesis (Figure 20B). In cells that

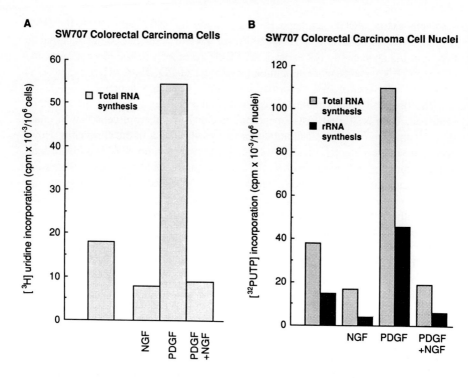

**FIGURE 20.**   Effect of NGF and PDGF on RNA synthesis in intact SW707 colorectal carcinoma cells (A) and in the nuclei isolated from these cells (B). SW707 cells express the cell surface receptors and the nuclear receptors for both NGF and PDGF. Cells were incubated 24 h with NGF (10 ng/ml) or PDGF (A, B; 10 ng/ml), or with both PDGF and NGF (A). Nuclei were incubated 1 h with [$^{32}$P]UTP.

express only PDGF receptor, but not NGF receptors, the effect of PDGF was not affected by NGF.[172]

Other growth factors, such as EGF, insulin, IGF-I (mixed with NGF or PDGF alone, or with both), and PDGF plus NGF, did not modulate the effect exerted by NGF and PDGF.[172]

Biological activity of the living cells is predominantly dependent on protein synthesis. In rapidly proliferating tumor cells, protein synthesis exhibits significantly high levels. Each factor which significantly blocks protein synthesis would, to a certain degree, arrest growth of tumor cells. Therefore, we suspected that inhibition of rRNA synthesis by 50% in cells exposed to NGF must affect assembly of ribosomes and decrease protein synthesis. In order to test this hypothesis, SW707 cells were exposed for 48 h to NGF, followed by 2 h incubation with [$^{35}$S]methionine. Protein synthesis, measured as [$^{35}$S]methionine incorporation into TCA-precipitable cell fraction, was lower by 60% in cells exposed to NGF than in cells not exposed to NGF (not shown). In contrast, when the same cells were exposed for 48 h to PDGF, protein synthesis was 65% higher than in cells not exposed to PDGF. When cells were exposed simultaneously to NGF and PDGF, protein synthesis was at a

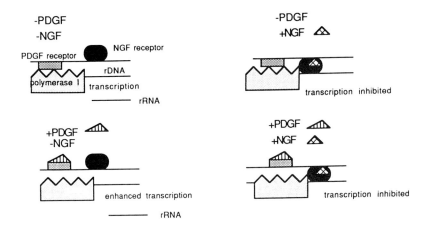

**FIGURE 21.** Hypothetical mechanism of PDGF and NGF effect on transcription of ribosomal DNA. Binding of PDGF to its chromatin receptor induces conformational changes which enhance transcription of ribosomal DNA by polymerase I. Binding of NGF to its chromatin receptor blocks binding of polymerase I to DNA, which inhibits transcription of ribosomal genes independently of the presence or absence of PDGF. (From Rakowicz-Szulczynska, E. M. and Koprowski, H., *Biochim. Biophys. Res. Commun.*, 163, 649, 1989. With permission.)

similar level as in the presence of NGF alone (approximately 60% lower than in cells not exposed to NGF or to PDGF). Thus NGF abolished the stimulatory effect of PDGF on protein synthesis.[172]

Analysis of SW707 cell growth in the absence or presence of NGF or PDGF, or both growth factors, indicated that PDGF alone stimulated significant growth of these cells (by more than 100%). However, in the presence of 10 ng/ml NGF, tumor cell growth was inhibited to the level of 54%, i.e., to the level of growth observed in the presence of 10 ng/ml NGF alone (Table 9). After mixing only 5 ng of NGF with 10 ng/ml of PDGF, DNA synthesis was inhibited to 64%. Even 1 ng/ml of NGF was able to antagonize the effect of PDGF; proliferation was the same as in the absence of these growth factors. The results indicate that NGF is a very potent inhibitor of tumor cell growth.

Since both NGF and PDGF recognize different nuclear receptors, but both affect rRNA synthesis, a simple model of rRNA synthesis regulated by these growth factors was described (Figure 21).[172] Since rRNA synthesis occurs efficiently in the absence of PDGF, we suggest that PDGF, after binding to the specific nuclear receptor, induces conformational changes which only enhance transcription of rDNA. In contrast, NGF, after binding to its chromatin receptor, induces conformational changes which make polymerase I binding to the DNA less efficient. In consequence, NGF abolishes the stimulatory effect of PDGF.[172]

In several control experiments described before,[172] we found that NGF and PDGF affect rRNA synthesis only in those cells in which specific nuclear receptors are expressed. Thus, NGF and PDGF probably specifically affect transcription of rDNA by binding to the chromatin proteins specific for the target cells rather than interacting with polymerase I, which is present in the nuclei of all cell lines. The fact that NGF, by binding to a specific chromatin receptor, may abolish the effect of PDGF, which is known to be one of the basic growth factors which promote tumor cell growth, sheds a new light on NGF function in tumor and normal cells. Since the nuclear receptor is critical for the inhibitory effect of NGF, we may risk a hypothesis, that the NGF chromatin receptor represents an anti-proliferative, anti-oncogenic product. The studies described in the next chapters would further attract this hypothesis.

## H. CELL RESPONSE TO NGF IN THE ABSENCE OF THE CHROMATIN RECEPTOR OR PRESENCE OF AN "INACTIVE" CHROMATIN RECEPTOR

In the sections above, we documented that NGF translocated to the nucleus of intact cells, or into the isolated nucleus in a cell-free system, binds to the 230,000-$M_r$ chromatin receptor typical for melanoma cells,[171,210] or to the 35,000-$M_r$ chromatin receptor typical to colorectal carcinoma cells,[171,176] which leads to inhibition of rRNA synthesis.

In breast carcinoma cell line SKBr 5, which expresses mainly the 90,000-$M_r$ chromatin receptor, and, in much smaller quantities, the dimeric 210,000-$M_r$ receptor, NGF was effectively internalized and translocated to the nucleus, but did not affect RNA synthesis.[212] In intact SKBr 5 cells, RNA synthesis increased by 10% in the presence of NGF (Figure 22A), but was unaffected after exposure to NGF of the isolated nuclei (Figure 22B). The response of SKBr 5 cells to NGF was similar to that of WM164 melanoma cells which do not express chromatin receptor for NGF and do not bind NGF to the chromatin.[212] In A875 cells which express the 230,000-$M_r$ chromatin receptor, both RNA synthesis in intact cells and RNA/rRNA synthesis in isolated nuclei were affected by NGF. We suggest that interaction of NGF with the 230,000-$M_r$ structure of the melanoma cell chromatin receptor is critical for inhibition of rRNA synthesis.

Analysis of cell growth response to NGF indicated that SKBr 5 and WM164 cells exposed to increasing concentrations of NGF (5 to 40 ng) responded by progressively increasing uptake of [$^3$H]thymidine into DNA (Figure 23). In contrast, A875 melanoma cells that express the 230,000-$M_r$ receptor responded to NGF by inhibiting [$^3$H]thymidine incorporation. The results indicate that binding of NGF to the chromatin of the target cells is critical but not sufficient to exert inhibitory effect on rRNA synthesis and, in consequence, on cell proliferation. It seems that different molecular forms of the chromatin receptor exist which make the molecular mechanism of NGF action more complicated. We have analyzed an expression of a one-gene family, those for rRNA, since rRNA is expressed in abundant quantities, which makes the fluctuation in synthesis easy to detect. However, it is likely that several unique genes may be regulated after NGF binds to a specific chromatin receptor. Whether different molecular forms of the chromatin receptor mediate unique effects of NGF on gene regulation level remains to be established.

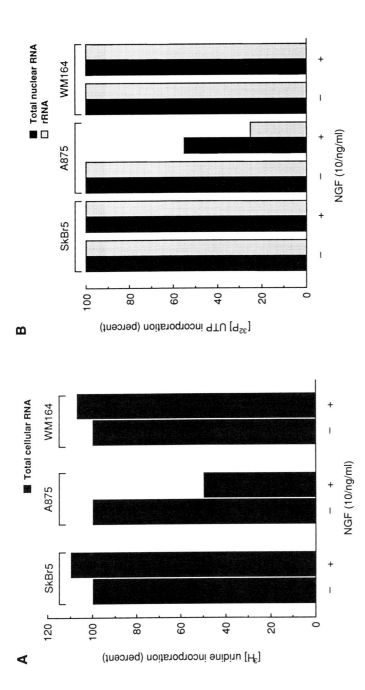

**FIGURE 22.** (A) RNA synthesis in intact SKBr 5 breast carcinoma cells and WM164 and A875 melanoma cells after 24 h incubation with [5,6-³H]uridine (100 μCi/ml; sp. act. 48 Ci/mmol; Amersham) in the absence (−) or presence (+) of NGF (10 ng/ml). (B) RNA and rRNA synthesis in nuclei isolated from SKBr 5 breast carcinoma cells and WM164 and A875 melanoma cells, incubated 1 h with [³²P]UTP in the absence (−) or presence (+) of NGF (10 ng/ml). (From Rakowicz-Szulczynska, E.M., *J. Cell Physiol.*, 154, 71, 1992. With permission.)

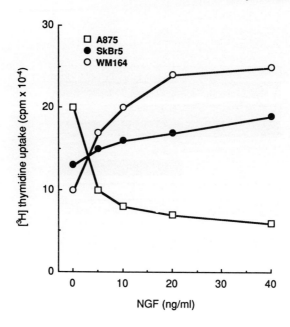

**FIGURE 23.**   Cell growth response to NGF. SKBr 5 breast carcinoma cells (which express a 90,000-$M_r$ chromatin receptor), A875 melanoma cells (230,000-$M_r$ chromatin receptor), and WM164 cells (do not express chromatin receptor) were exposed for 4 d to NGF in the presence of [6-³H]thymidine (added daily; 10 μCi/ml, sp. act. 24 Ci/mmol; Amersham). (From Rakowicz-Szulczynska, E. M., *J. Cell Physiol.*, 154, 71, 1992. With permission.)

# IV. IS THE CELL RESPONSE TO NGF REGULATED BY TWO INDEPENDENT RECEPTORS?

The possibility that a specific growth factor may activate, as well as inhibit, cell growth through the single mechanism that involves binding of the growth factor to the cell surface receptor and induction of second messengers, did not find experimental confirmation. Our studies indicate that in addition to the cell surface receptor, another receptor is located in the chromatin. In the case of NGF, both receptors seem to exhibit opposite functions, i.e., the cell surface receptor mediates the activatory effect of NGF, while the nuclear receptor mediates the inhibitory effect. We suggest that the cell growth response depends on the ratio between the cell surface and the nuclear receptor, instead of being directly dependent on the number of the cell surface receptors. The model experiments described below support this hypothesis.

## A. INDUCTION OF THE CHROMATIN RECEPTOR BY NGF

In cells that express both the cell surface and the chromatin receptor, the function of one of these receptors cannot be separated from the other, unless the nuclei are isolated. An ideal model system for studies on the function of each of these receptors provide melanoma cell line WM164 cells, which, growing in the absence of NGF

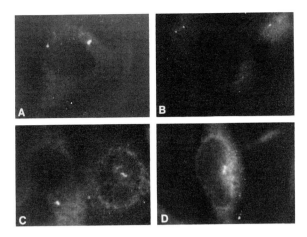

**FIGURE 24.** Immunofluorescence detection of internalized NGF. Indirect immunofluorescence staining of WM164 melanoma cells (A, B) and of WM164 cells transfected with cDNA for NGF cell surface receptor (TrWM164) (C, D). (A) and (B), and (C) and (D) are duplicates from independent experiments. Cells were incubated 24 h with NGF (10 ng/ml) followed by incubation with rabbit anti-NGF serum and fluoresceine-conjugated sheep anti-rabbit IgG.

in the medium, do not express the chromatin receptor, but do express a low level of the cell surface receptor.[174] After exposure to NGF, WM164 cells begin to express the chromatin receptor in addition to the cell surface receptor.[174]

WM164 melanoma cells after 24-h incubation with NGF showed weak indirect immunofluorescence staining of the cytoplasm with rabbit anti-NGF IgG (Figure 24A and B). Low internalization of NGF correlated with the low expression of the NGF cell-surface receptor. The lack of nuclear fluorescence suggests that NGF does not bind to the chromatin of these cells (chromatin receptor is not expressed). In cell fractionation studies (Table 9), WM164 cells, incubated for 24 h with [125]I-NGF, exhibited low internalization of [125]I-NGF, with strictly cytoplasmic localization.[174]

To test the possibility that total uptake of [125]I-NGF by WM164 cells was too low to indicate nuclear translocation, WM164 cells were transfected with cDNA for the NGF cell surface receptor.[174] Both WM164 cells (Figure 24A and B) and the cells of the transfected cell line (TrWM164 cells) showed strong fluorescence staining of the cytoplasm and of the perinuclear region (Figure 24C and D), but not of the nucleus. Strictly cytoplasmic localization of NGF in WM164 and TrWM164 cells was confirmed by fractionation of cells incubated 24 h with [125]I-NGF (Table 10). Nuclear binding of [125]I-NGF was not above the background level in these cells.

The fact that the transfected cells showed more of [125]I-NGF molecules in the cytoplasm, but not in the chromatin, strongly suggests that nuclear accumulation does not parallel cytoplasmic accumulation of NGF. Instead, binding of NGF to the chromatin requires a specific chromatin receptor that represents a molecule different from the cell-surface receptor. When the time of incubation of WM164

TABLE 9
Effect of NGF and PDGF
on Proliferation of SW707
Colorectal Carcinoma Cells

| NGF (ng/ml) | PDGF (ng/ml) | [³H]thymidine incorporation | |
|---|---|---|---|
| | | cpm | % |
| 0 | 0 | 70,000 | 100 |
| 10 | 0 | 36,000 | 50 |
| 0 | 10 | 150,000 | 214 |
| 10 | 10 | 38,000 | 54 |
| 5 | 10 | 45,000 | 64 |
| 1 | 10 | 70,500 | 100 |

TABLE 10
Nuclear Accumulation of ¹²⁵I-NGF in Cells not Exposed
and Exposed to NGF (24 h of Incubation)

| Cell line | ¹²⁵I-NGF (cpm per cell)[a] | | | |
|---|---|---|---|---|
| | Cytoplasm | Nuclear membrane | Nucleoplasm | Chromatin |
| WM164 | 1,820 | 100 | 30 | 30 |
| WM164/NGF[b] | 2,000 | 98 | 10 | 60 |
| TrWM164[c] | 3,000 | 110 | 38 | 25 |
| TrWM164/NGF[b] | 4,280 | 100 | 120 | 1,200 |

[a]  Experiments were performed in duplicate (SD < 10%).
[b]  WM164/NGF and TrWM164/NGF were exposed for 10 d to NGF (10 ng/ml).
[c]  TrWM164 cells are WM164 melanoma cells (express low level of the NGF cell surface receptor) which were transfected with cDNA for the cell surface receptor.

From Rakowicz-Szulczynska, E. M., Reddy, U., Vorbrodt, A., Herlyn, D., and Koprowski, H., *Mol. Carcinogen.*, 4, 388, 1991. With permission.

and TrWM164 cells was decreased from 24 h to 1 h, a low level of ¹²⁵I-NGF was detected in the nucleus. However, after chromatin purification, no chromatin-bound ¹²⁵I-NGF was detected. The latest results indicate that even if ¹²⁵I-NGF penetrates the nucleus of these cells, in the absence of a specific chromatin receptor, it is not bound to the chromatin and is rapidly degraded (not shown).

To determine whether unlabeled NGF is able to stimulate expression of NGF receptor in WM164 and TrWM164 cells, as NGF does in A875 or SW707 cells (see Table 2), we exposed both cell lines for 10 d to NGF (10 ng/ml). Cells exposed to NGF began to accumulate NGF in the nucleus (chromatin) (Table 9).

**TABLE 11**

## Effect of NGF on [³H]uridine Incorporation into RNA Synthesized in Intact Cells (Experiment A, 24 h Incubation) and on Incorporation of [³²P]UTP into Total and Ribosomal RNA Synthesized in Isolated Nuclei (Experiment B, 1 h Incubation)

| Cell line | NGF (5 ng/ml) | Experiment A [³H]uridine incorporation[a] (cpm/10⁶ cells) | Experiment B [³²P]UTP incorporation[b] (cpm/10⁶ nuclei) | [³²P]UTP RNA hybridization to rDNA[c] (cpm) |
|---|---|---|---|---|
| WM164 | −[f] | 45,000 | 36,500 | 15,200 |
| | + | 48,000 | 36,750 | 15,450 |
| TrWM164[d] | − | 50,000 | 37,000 | 16,500 |
| | + | 56,000 | 37,100 | 16,750 |
| WM164/NGF[e] | − | 45,500 | 36,000 | 15,500 |
| | + | 40,000 | 22,000 | 10,000 |
| TrWM164/NGF[e] | − | 51,000 | 36,900 | 16,850 |
| | + | 42,000 | 16,000 | 8,300 |

[a,b,c] Data shows a representative series of experiments: the SD of the mean value for four independent series of experiments did not exceed 12% in [a], 17% in [b], and 15% in [c].

[d] TrWM164 cells are WM164 cells transfected with cDNA for the cell surface NGF receptor.

[e] WM164/NGF and TrWM164/NGF were cells exposed for 10 d to NGF (10 ng/ml).

[f] Second exposure to NGF ( + ); control experiment where no NGF was added ( − ).

To determine how WM164 and TrWM164, which express only the cell surface receptor, respond to NGF, both cell lines were exposed to [³H]uridine (24-h exposure) or [³H]thymidine (4-d exposure) in the presence or absence of NGF.

In both WM164 and TrWM164 cells, NGF stimulated RNA synthesis[174] (Table 11). Growth of both cell lines was also stimulated by NGF (Figure 25). The activatory effect of NGF was higher in TrWM164 cells, which suggests a correlation with the number of the cell surface receptors.

To establish the long-term effect of NGF on the RNA synthesis and growth of melanoma cells that do not accumulate NGF in the nucleus, WM164 cells and TrWM164 cells were grown for 10 d in the presence of 10 ng/ml of NGF (first exposure).[174] After 10 d, the cultures were washed and seeded for 24 h in a fresh medium containing [³H]uridine, or for 4 d in the medium with [³H]thymidine and different concentrations of NGF (second exposure).

In cells pre-exposed to NGF, [³H]uridine incorporation into RNA in the presence of NGF was lower than in its absence. The second exposure of WM164 and TrWM164 cells to NGF, depending on NGF concentration, did not affect cell proliferation, or it slightly inhibited the growth of these cells (Figure 25).

Since WM164 and TrWM164 cells that were not preincubated for 10 d with NGF were stimulated to proliferate by NGF (Figure 25), it was likely that the 10-d exposure to NGF resulted in induction of the chromatin receptor for NGF.

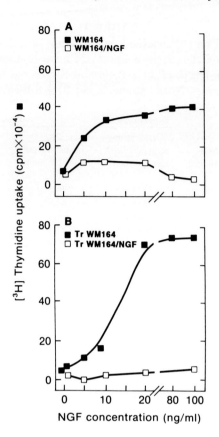

**FIGURE 25.** Effect of NGF on proliferation of WM164 cells and TrWM164 cells that express only the cell surface receptor (■), and on the same cells that were pre-exposed for 10 d to NGF and therefore express both the cell surface and the chromatin NGF receptors (□).

To determine whether these results could be explained by the direct binding of NGF to the chromatin observed in cells preexposed to NGF (Table 9), experiments were performed in a cell-free system. NGF was without any effect on RNA or rRNA synthesis in nuclei from WM164 and TrWM164 cells not exposed to NGF, but NGF inhibited both RNA and rRNA synthesis in nuclei from cells exposed for 10 d to NGF (Table 10). The results presented strongly suggest that the switch of activatory to inhibitory action of NGF must be mediated by an induced chromatin receptor to which it binds.

## 1. Identification of the NGF Chromatin Receptor Induced by NGF in WM164 and TrWM164 Cells

WM164 and TrWM164 cells not preincubated, or preincubated for 10 d with NGF as above, were labeled with [35S]methionine in two lots. In one lot, the cultures were labeled in the fresh medium only, and in the other the cells were labeled at

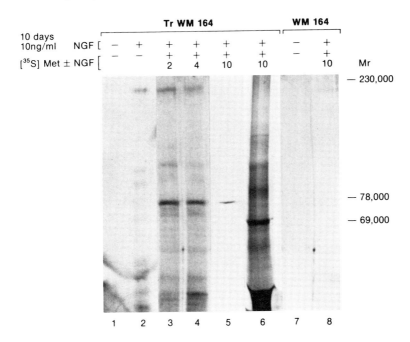

**FIGURE 26.** Autoradiographic detection of NGF chromatin receptor and cell-surface receptor. SDS-7.5% PAGE of [$^{35}$S]methionine-labeled chromatin (lanes 1 to 5) and cell-surface membrane (lane 6) proteins immunoprecipitated from TrWM164 cell or WM164 cell chromatin (lanes 7 and 8) before (lanes 1 and 7) or after (lanes 2 to 6 and 8) 10 d of preincubation with NGF (10 ng/ml). Cells were exposed for 18 h to [$^3$H]methionine alone (lanes 1, 2, and 7) or to the indicated concentrations (in ng/ml) of NGF (lanes 3 to 6 and 8). (From Rakowicz-Szulczynska, E. M., Reddy, U., Vorbrodt, A., Herlyn, D., and Koprowski, H., *Mol. Carcinogen.*, 4, 388, copyright © 1991. With permission of Wiley-Liss, division of John Wiley and Sons, Inc.)

the time of the second exposure to NGF. After 18 h of labeling with [$^{35}$S]methionine, the chromatin was isolated, digested with *Eco*RI, and precipitated with mAb ME 20.4, directed against the NGF cell-surface receptor, as described previously.[210] No protein was immunoprecipitated from TrWM164 (Figure 26, lane 1) or WM164 cells (Figure 26, lane 7) not exposed to NGF, which correlates with the observation described above that these cells do not accumulate NGF in the nucleus. A [$^{35}$S]methionine-labeled protein of high $M_r$ (230,000) was precipitated by the mAb from the chromatin of TrWM164 cells after a single 10 d exposure of those cells to NGF[174] (Figure 26, lane 2). From the chromatin of TrWM164 cells labeled with [$^{35}$S]methionine in the presence of NGF, in addition to the 230,000-$M_r$ protein, a protein of lower $M_r$ (78,000) was precipitated (Figure 26, lanes 3 and 4). Only the 78,000-$M_r$ band was visible when cells were labeled with [$^{35}$S]methionine in the presence of the highest (10 ng/ml) concentration of NGF[174] (Figure 26, lane 5).

From the chromatin of WM164 cells, mAb ME 20.4 precipitated only a [$^{35}$S]methionine-labeled 230,000-$M_r$ protein, regardless of exposure of cells to NGF

(Figure 26, lane 8). The 230,000-$M_r$ band was much weaker than in the TrWM164 cells. This seems to indicate that the 230,000-$M_r$ chromatin receptor typical for melanoma lineages was induced during the 10-d exposure to NGF.

To eliminate the possibility that the 78,000-$M_r$ chromatin protein in fact represented a cell surface receptor translocated to the nucleus together with NGF, the cell surface membrane fraction was also immunoprecipitated with mAb ME 20.4. The immunoprecipitated cell surface receptor exhibited a $M_r$ of 69,000 (Figure 26, lane 6), which suggests that the 78,000-$M_r$ chromatin protein was different from the cell surface receptor. It is likely that the 78,000-$M_r$ protein represents a subunit corresponding to the 90,000-$M_r$ subunit dissociating from the melanoma 451 line 230,000-$M_r$ receptor in the presence of NGF (Figure 6).

mAb ME 20.4 did not precipitate any protein from the chromatin of cells labeled with [$^{35}$S]cysteine, regardless of their treatment (data not shown). Since cysteine is an amino acid characteristic for the cell surface receptor (see Table 5), these results seem to further eliminate the surface origin of the protein immunoprecipitated from the chromatin.

The electrophoretic mobility and the diffuse shape of the high-$M_r$ protein induced by NGF in chromatin of TrWM164 cells (Figure 26) were the same as that of the protein expressed in the chromatin of metastatic melanoma cell lines (Figures 5 and 6).

The results obtained clearly indicate that NGF induces expression of the NGF chromatin receptor which switches the stimulatory effect of NGF on cell growth to inhibitory. Thus, NGF activates cell growth by binding to the cell surface receptor. In the absence of the nuclear receptor, this is the only effect of NGF observed in WM164 cells. After transfection of WM164 cells with cDNA for the cell surface NGF receptor, the expression of the cell surface receptor increased, which resulted in much higher growth response to NGF, compared to non-transfected cells. When long exposure to NGF resulted in induction of the 230,000-$M_r$ chromatin receptor, NGF was bound to the chromatin and affected rRNA synthesis. Consequently, the cell surface receptor-mediated stimulatory action of NGF was abolished. Thus the nuclear (chromatin) receptor for NGF acts as a strong inhibitor of cell growth. The experiments suggest that melanoma cells growth response to NGF is regulated by two independent mechanisms: the cell surface receptor-mediated mechanism and the chromatin receptor-mediated mechanism.

## B. INDUCTION OF THE CHROMATIN RECEPTOR BY GAMMA-INTERFERON

Interferons (IFN), known compounds of antiviral and immunomodulatory activity,[250] exert an inhibitory effect on the growth of some transplantable tumors in mice and metastatic tumors in humans.[251-253] Gamma-interferon ($\gamma$-IFN) and $\beta$-IFN suppress development of human bladder papillomas or carcinoma *in situ*[251] and protect against chemical carcinogenesis.[252] IFN affect cell proliferation and differentiation[254,255] by yet unknown molecular mechanisms. It is accepted that IFN modulate gene expression on transcriptional and translational levels.[250,255-257] IFN

## TABLE 12
### Internalization and Nuclear Uptake of $^{125}$I-NGF in Tumor Cells Exposed or not Exposed to $\gamma$-IFN

| | | Molecules/cell[a] | | | |
|---|---|---|---|---|---|
| Cell lines | $\gamma$-IFN | Cytoplasm | Nucleoplasm | Nuclear membranes | Chromatin |
| *Melanoma* | | | | | |
| HS294 | – | 45,000 | 750 | 120 | 3,800 |
| | + | 13,200 | 250 | 75 | 695 |
| WM164 | – | 1,600 | 15 | 10 | 30 |
| | + | 650 | 12 | 8 | 30 |
| *Breast carcinoma* | | | | | |
| SKBr 5 | – | 9,000 | 650 | 220 | 29,000 |
| | + | 6,400 | 700 | 200 | 1,600 |
| *Colorectal Carcinoma* | | | | | |
| SW707 | – | 800 | 55 | 10 | 1,405 |
| | + | 1,200 | 150 | 17 | 3,014 |
| SW1116 | – | *n.d.*[b] | *n.d.* | *n.d.* | *n.d.* |
| | + | 1,000 | 100 | 12 | 2,500 |

*Note:* Cells were incubated for 24 h with $^{125}$I-NGF (10 ng/ml) in the presence (+) or absence (−) of $\gamma$-IFN at a concentration of 1000 units/ml.

[a] Calculation of molecules per one cell; mean from three experiments; SD = 5% for the cells not exposed to $\gamma$-IFN and 10 to 15% for the cells exposed to $\gamma$-IFN.

[b] *n.d.*, not detectable.

were found to modulate activity of at least 100 different genes. A common consensus element has been identified in the 5′ regions of most IFN-regulated genes.[258,259]

IFN induce expression of 18 genes up to 40-fold in T98 neuroblastoma cells.[256] In Ehrlich ascites tumor cells[260] or in BALB/c-3T3 cells,[261] IFN inhibit secretion of some proteins and induce secretion of others. Stamenkovic et al.[262] reported that in B cells and epithelial neoplasms, $\gamma$-IFN induces a surface molecule, Bp50, which shows homology to the NGF receptor. We have found that $\gamma$-IFN modulates expression of NGF receptors in several tumor cell lines.[176]

Melanoma, breast carcinoma, and colorectal carcinoma cell lines that express the cell surface and the chromatin receptors for NGF were exposed for 24 h to $^{125}$I-NGF, in the absence or presence of $\gamma$-IFN (1000 units/ml) (Table 12). In the presence of $\gamma$-IFN, internalization and nuclear uptake of $^{125}$I-NGF decreased in melanoma and breast carcinoma cells, but increased in colorectal carcinoma SW707 cell lines, compared to cells not exposed to $\gamma$-IFN.[176] We suspected that in melanoma and breast carcinoma cells, $\gamma$-IFN inhibited, while in SW707 colorectal carcinoma cells, $\gamma$-IFN stimulated, expression of the receptors for NGF. To determine whether $\gamma$-IFN is able to induce *de novo* synthesis of NGF receptors, colorectal carcinoma cell line SW1116, which does not express NGF receptors, was exposed to $^{125}$I-NGF in the absence or presence of $\gamma$-IFN. SW1116 cells not exposed to $\gamma$-IFN did not

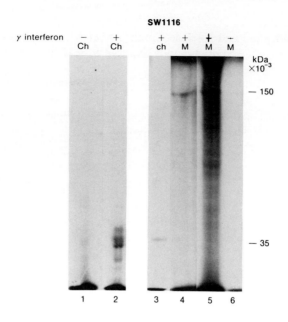

**FIGURE 27.** Autoradiographic detection of electrophoretically separated proteins immunoprecipitated from cell membranes and from chromatin of cells exposed or not exposed to γ-IFN. [$^{35}$S]methionine-labeled proteins were immunoprecipitated with mAb 20.4 against NGF receptor from cell membranes (M) or from chromatin (Ch) of SW1116 cells exposed (+) or not exposed (−) to γ-IFN. Cells were exposed to 1000 units of γ-IFN/ml (lanes 2 and 5), 500 units/ml (lanes 3 and 4). Electrophoresis was performed in 7.5% polyacrylamide gel with 0.1% SDS. Each immunoprecipitate originated from 2 × 10$^7$ cells.

internalize $^{125}$I-NGF, but did internalize when incubated with $^{125}$I-NGF in the presence of γ-IFN (Table 12). The internalized $^{125}$I-NGF was localized in the cytoplasm and in the nucleus of SW1116 cells, which suggested that both the cell surface and the nuclear receptors were expressed in γ-IFN treated SW1116 colorectal carcinoma cells.

To determine whether γ-IFN induced expression of NGF receptors, or, alternatively, activated uptake of $^{125}$I-NGF in the receptor-independent way, cell membranes and the chromatin obtained from SW1116 and SW707 colorectal carcinoma cells were exposed for 24 h to γ-IFN in the presence of [$^{35}$S]methionine, then immunoprecipitated with mAb 20.4 against the NGF receptor (Figure 27).

Immunoprecipitation with mAb ME 20.4 of the cell surface membranes and of the *Eco*RI-digested chromatin from SW1116 cells not exposed to γ-IFN revealed no protein (Figure 27, lanes 1 and 6). From cells exposed to γ-IFN, a 150,000-$M_r$ cell membrane protein (Figure 27, lanes 4 and 5) and a 35,000-$M_r$ chromatin protein (Figure 27, lanes 2 and 3) were immunoprecipitated.[176] A lower concentrations of γ-IFN (500 units/ml) induced lower expression of both receptors (Figure 27, lanes 3 and 4) than the higher concentration (100 units/ml) (Figure 27, lanes 2 and 5).

The molecular weights of the cell surface and the chromatin receptors induced by γ-IFN in SW1116 colorectal carcinoma cells correlated with the molecular weight of receptors identified in SW707 colorectal carcinoma cells (Figure 11). The results obtained suggest that γ-IFN induces expression of the cell surface and the chromatin receptor for NGF in the colorectal carcinoma SW1116 cell line which does not express these receptors before γ-IFN exposure.

## 1. Effect of γ-IFN on NGF-Dependent Synthesis of Ribosomal RNA and Cell Proliferation

SW1116 cells exposed to γ-IFN for 24 h, and then exposed to NGF for 1 h or 24 h, showed 30 and 40% lower RNA synthesis, respectively, than SW1116 cells not exposed to γ-IFN (Table 13). In SW707 cells exposed or not exposed to γ-IFN, RNA synthesis decreased by 40% after incubation with NGF. γ-IFN alone did not change RNA synthesis in these cells.[176]

In order to establish whether the γ-IFN-induced chromatin receptor in SW1116 colorectal carcinoma cells mediates an inhibitory effect of NGF on rRNA synthesis as does the chromatin receptor in SW707 cells,[172] NGF-dependent RNA synthesis was measured in isolated nuclei. In nuclei isolated from SW1116 cells exposed to γ-IFN, NGF inhibited rRNA synthesis by 52% but had no effect on rRNA synthesis in nuclei isolated from cells not exposed to γ-IFN (Table 13). In nuclei isolated from SW707 cells either exposed or not exposed to γ-IFN, rRNA synthesis was inhibited by 66%.[176]

Analysis of the growth response to NGF of SW1116 cells, in which γ-IFN induced the chromatin receptor for NGF, indicated 25% lower [³H]thymidine incorporation into DNA of cells exposed to 500 units/ml of γ-IFN, and 50% lower incorporation into DNA of cells exposed to 1000 units/ml of γ-IFN, than that of cells not exposed to γ-IFN (not shown). The results we obtained suggest that the chromatin receptor for NGF, induced in SW1116 cells by γ-IFN, mediates the inhibitory action of NGF on rRNA synthesis and leads to the inhibition of tumor cell growth. In SW707 cells, γ-IFN enhanced the already inhibitory effect of NGF (Table 14).

## 2. Effect of γ-IFN on Chromatin Protein Synthesis in Colorectal Carcinoma Cells

To establish whether the chromatin receptor for NGF represents the only protein with expression regulated by γ-IFN in colorectal carcinoma cells, the SW1116 and SW707 cells were labeled with [³⁵S]methionine in the presence or absence of γ-IFN (1000 units/ml). Chromatin proteins were isolated and analyzed by two-dimensional gel electrophoresis[176] (Figure 28). In SW1116 cells, exposure to γ-IFN resulted in quantitative changes of a minor fraction of chromatin proteins (Figure 28A and B). Significant variations in the chromatin protein composition were observed between the SW707 colorectal cells exposed (Figure 28D) and not exposed (Figure 28C) to γ-IFN. Some chromatin protein expressed in the chromatin of cells not exposed to γ-IFN were expressed at very low levels in cells exposed to γ-IFN and vice versa, several chromatin proteins absent or present in very low quantities before exposure were expressed in significant amounts after exposure to γ-IFN. The results obtained indicate that in addition to the chromatin receptor for NGF,

**TABLE 13**

**Effect of NGF on RNA Synthesis in Cells Exposed and not Exposed to γ-IFN**

| Cell line | γ-IFN[a] | NGF | RNA synthesis in intact cells[b] [³H]uridine (cpm/10⁶ cells) | RNA synthesis inhibition | RNA synthesis in isolated nuclei[c] [³²P]UTP (cpm/10⁶ nuclei) | [³²P]UTP RNA hybridization to rDNA cpm | inhibition of rRNA synthesis (%)[d] |
|---|---|---|---|---|---|---|---|
| SW1116 | – | – | 17,500 | 0 | 40,500 | 18,000 | 0 |
| | – | + | 18,000 | 0 | 40,800 | 18,100 | 0 |
| | + | – | 17,400 | 0 | 38,000 | 17,500 | 0 |
| | + | + | 12,000 | 30 | 21,400 | 8,500 | 50 |
| SW707 | – | – | 14,200 | 0 | 36,000 | 15,200 | 0 |
| | – | + | 8,500 | 40 | 24,700 | 5,500 | 75 |
| | + | – | 14,000 | 0 | 34,500 | 14,950 | 0 |
| | + | + | 8,250 | 40 | 21,000 | 5,200 | 75 |

[a]   –, cells not exposed; +, cells exposed to γ-IFN.

[b]   Cells were exposed for 24 h or not exposed to γ-IFN (1000 units/ml) before being incubated with NGF (10 ng/ml) and [³H]uridine for 1 h or 24 h; SD from three experiments, 7 to 16%.

[c]   Nuclei were isolated from cells not exposed to γ-IFN or exposed to γ-IFN for 24 h and incubated for 1 h with [³²P]UTP in the presence or absence of NGF (10 ng/ml). Representative data from one experiment; SD from four experiments were 13 to 17%.

[d]   Inhibition of hybridization corresponds to inhibition of rRNA synthesis.

**TABLE 14**

**Effect of NGF on Proliferation of SW1116 and
SW707 Colorectal Carcinoma Cells
Exposed or not Exposed to γ-IFN[a]**

| Cell line | γ-IFN | NGF | [³H]thymidine incorporation | |
| --- | --- | --- | --- | --- |
| | | | cpm | % |
| SW1116 | − | − | 24,000 | 100 |
| | − | + | 24,200 | 100 |
| | + (500 u/ml) | + | 18,000 | 75 |
| | + (1000 u/ml) | + | 13,000 | 53 |
| | + (1000 u/ml) | − | 24,500 | 100 |
| SW707 | − | − | 23,000 | 100 |
| | − | + | 11,500 | 50 |
| | + (500 u/ml) | + | 10,200 | 44 |
| | + (1000 u/ml) | + | 8,900 | 39 |
| | + (1000 u/ml) | − | 23,100 | 100 |

*Note:* 2 × 10⁶ cells were incubated for 5 d with [³H]thymidine in the
presence or absence of γ-IFN (500 or 1000 units/ml) and/or NGF
(10 ng/ml).

[a] Representative data from one experiment; SD from three independent
experiments were below 10%.

the expression of several other chromatin proteins is modulated by cell exposure
to γ-IFN.[176] Those proteins, whose function is not yet established, may significantly
change transcription and/or replication of colorectal carcinoma cells.

### 3. Conclusions

Our results indicate that γ-IFN exerts a strong effect on both quantitative and
qualitative changes in the composition of nonhistone chromatin proteins. Among
others, γ-IFN exerts a critical effect on expression of the cell surface and chromatin
receptors for NGF. The effect is different in different tumor cell lines; in melanoma
and breast carcinoma cell lines, expression of NGF receptors significantly decreases
in the presence of γ-IFN. An opposite effect is exerted by γ-IFN in colorectal
carcinoma cells, where it stimulates or induces *de novo* synthesis of both the cell
surface and the chromatin receptors. In consequence, after NGF receptors are
induced, colorectal carcinoma cells respond to NGF by inhibiting growth. Inhibitory
effect is mediated by the chromatin receptor, which binds translocated to the nucleus
NGF, which consequently leads to inhibition of rRNA synthesis. The results indicate

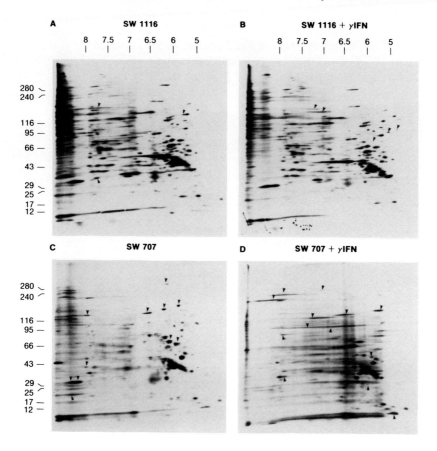

**FIGURE 28.** Analysis of chromatin proteins expressed in colorectal carcinoma cells exposed or not exposed to γ-IFN. 50μg of chromatin proteins isolated from SW1116 or SW707 cells labeled for 18 h with [$^{35}$S]methionine in the presence or absence of γ-IFN (500 units/ml) were subjected to two-dimensional gel electrophoresis. Each gel was incubated with enhancer, dried, and autoradiographed. Arrows indicate the position of proteins which showed changes in expression after exposure to γ-IFN. (From Rakowicz-Szulczynska, E. M. et al., *Growth Factors*, 6, 337, 1992. With permission.)

that γ-IFN by positive (as in colorectal carcinoma) or negative (in melanoma and breast carcinoma) regulation of the chromatin receptor may have a critical role in inhibiting the growth of some tumors, while promoting the growth of others.

## C. NGF CELL SURFACE TO CHROMATIN RECEPTOR RATIO-REGULATED GROWTH OF MELANOCYTES AND NEVUS CELLS *IN VITRO*

Normal skin melanocytes do not express, or express almost undetectable levels of, the NGF cell surface receptors.[263,264] During early passages in cell culture *in vitro*, human melanocytes growing in the presence of 12-0-tetradecanoylphorbol-13-acetate (TPA) began to express, on the cell surface, the NGF receptor and other

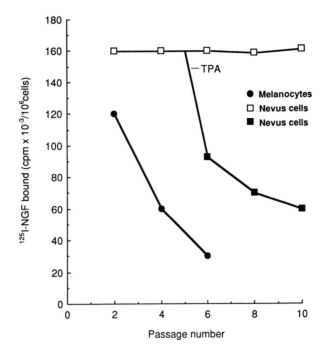

**FIGURE 29.** [125]I-NGF binding to the cell surface receptors expressed on melanocytes (●) and nevus cells (□, ■) *in vitro*. Binding of [125]I-NGF correlates with the expression of the surface receptors. Melanocytes were grown in the presence of TPA, and nevus cells in the presence (□) or absence (■) of TPA, and incubated with [125]I-NGF for 1 h at 0°C. Nonspecific binding of [125]I-NGF in the 100-fold excess of unlabeled NGF was subtracted. (From Rakowicz-Szulczynska, E. M. et al., *Growth Factors*, 6, 337, 1992. With permission.)

melanoma-associated antigens.[263] However, expression of the cell surface receptor for NGF decreases in the later passages of melanocytes.[263] NGF receptor is expressed on nevus cells, and TPA also stabilizes expression of NGF surface receptor on these cells.[265-268] Since NGF receptor is abundantly expressed on melanoma cells, it is likely that an increased expression of this receptor plays a role in malignant melanocytic tumors. We have tested whether the chromatin receptor plays a role in regulation of melanocyte and nevus cell growth.[211]

To monitor the expression of the cell surface receptors, melanocytes and nevus cells of different passages were incubated with [125]I-NGF (10 ng/ml) for 1 h at 0°C. At low temperature, endocytosis is inhibited and therefore [125]I-NGF binds to the cell surface receptor without internalization (Figure 29). The number of [125]I-NGF molecules bound to the cell surface of melanocytes was decreasing with the passage number, i.e., was highest in melanocytes at passage 2 and lowest at passage 6.[211] Nevus cells of all passages (4 to 10) bound the same number of [125]I-NGF molecules, which suggested that expression of the cell surface receptor was constant; however, when TPA was removed from the medium, cell surface binding of [125]I-NGF rapidly

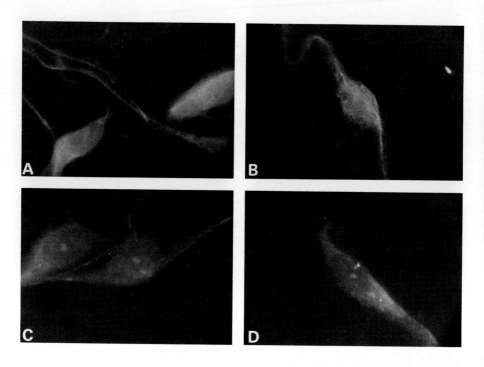

**FIGURE 30.** Indirect fluorescence staining of nevus cells (A, C) and of melanocytes (B, D) with anti-NGF rabbit serum. Nevus cells growing in the presence of TPA-passage 6 (A) or in the absence of TPA-passage 6 (C) and melanocytes growing in the presence of TPA of passage 2 (B) and passage 6 (D) were exposed to NGF (10 ng/ml) for 24 h. (From Rakowicz-Szulczynska, E. M., *J. Biol. Reg. Homeostatic Agents,* 6, 21, 1992. With permission of Wichtig Editore.)

decreased (Figure 29). In further experiments, we tested how melanocytes and nevus cells, which express different levels of the cell surface receptor, respond to NGF.

Intracellular localization of NGF was tested by indirect immunofluorescence staining of cells that had been preincubated 24 h with NGF with rabbit anti-NGF serum (Figure 30) and by fractionation of cells incubated with [125]I-NGF (Table 12).[211]

Melanocytes of the second or third passages, which express a high number of NGF surface receptors (Figure 29), showed strong intracellular fluorescence (Figure 30B). The intensity of fluorescence did not allow distinguishing the cytoplasmic fluorescence from the nuclear. In passages 5 to 6, which expressed lower levels of NGF surface receptors (Figure 30D), fluorescence of the cytoplasm was much weaker, and the nuclear fluorescence was well defined. Significantly higher density of fluorescence was observed in the nucleolus (Figure 30D).

Nevus cells growing in the presence of TPA showed strong intracellular fluorescence in passages 1 to 10 (Figure 30A). However, two weeks after TPA was removed from the medium when the cells were losing expression of the NGF surface

## TABLE 15
### Intracellular Distribution of [125]I-NGF
### in Melanocytes and Nevus Cells

| Cells | Passage | TPA | [125]I-NGF molecules/cell | | n/c NGF[a] |
|-------|---------|-----|-----------|-----------|-----------|
| | | | Cytoplasm | Chromatin | |
| Melanocytes | 2 | + | 25,715 | 4,476 | 0.15 |
| | 4 | + | 10,900 | 4,650 | 0.28 |
| | 6 | + | 5,200 | 4,600 | 0.88 |
| Nevus | 4 — 10 | + | 30,350 | 5,510 | 0.18 |
| | 6[b] | — | 13,250 | 5,610 | 0.42 |

[a]  Ratio of chromatin-bound to total internalized NGF.
[b]  Nevus cells growing in passages 1 to 5 in the presence of TPA were
incubated at passage 6 in the absence of TPA.

From Rakowicz-Szulczynska, E. M., *J. Biol. Reg. Homeostatic Agents*, 6,
21, 1992. With permission of Wichtig Editore.

receptor, the intracellular fluorescence of cytoplasm became weaker, and the fluorescence of the nucleus (nucleolus) stronger[211] (Figure 30C).

We suggest that the early strong fluorescence of the cytoplasm may have masked the fluorescence of the nucleus, which became visible after the fluorescence of cytoplasm weakened.

The intracellular distribution of [125]I-NGF in melanocytes and nevus cells (Table 15) correlated with the distribution of the fluorescence (Figure 30). In all passages of melanocytes, the amount of chromatin-bound [125]I-NGF was constant (Table 15). In the cytoplasm, the amount of NGF changed from a high of 25,715 molecules per cell during the early passages to a low of 5200 molecules per cell in the late passages. The amount of NGF accumulated in the cytoplasm correlates with the amount of NGF internalized by the cell, which in turn had depended on the expression of the cell surface NGF receptor. The changes in the ratio of the nuclear (chromatin-bound) to total intracellular NGF (n/c NGF) shown in Table 12 reflect changes in the ratio of chromatin and cell surface receptors.[211]

In nevus cells growing in the presence of TPA, the n/c NGF ratio was low and constant (0.18). After removal of TPA from the medium, the n/c NGF ratio increased to 0.42 because the amount of [125]I-NGF internalized by the cell dropped without changing the amount of nuclear NGF.

The results show that TPA stimulates expression of the cell surface receptor for NGF but not of the chromatin receptor which is expressed at a constant level in melanocytes and nevus cells *in vitro*.[211]

### 1. Identification of the Chromatin Receptor in Melanocytes

Chromatin isolated from melanocytes proliferating *in vitro* in the presence of TPA and [[35]S]methionine was digested with *Eco*RI and immunoprecipitated with

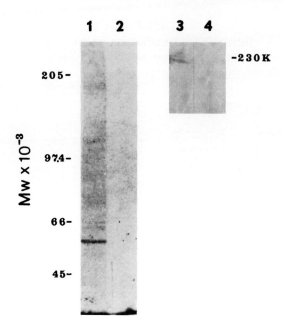

**FIGURE 31.** SDS-PAGE (7.5% polyacrylamide gel) of [³⁵S]methionine-labeled chromatin protein from melanocytes proliferating in the presence of TPA (lanes 1 and 2), intact (lane 1), and *Eco*RI-digested (lane 2) chromatin, and of chromatin protein immunoprecipitated from *Eco*RI-digested chromatin with mAb ME 20.4 against NGF receptor (lane 3), or with nonspecific antibody P3 × 63Ag8 (lane 4). Lanes 1 and 2, autoradiographic exposure; lanes 3 and 4, Coomassie blue staining. (From Rakowicz-Szulczynska, E. M., Herlyn, M., and Koprowski, H., *Cancer Res.*, 48, 7200, 1988. With permission of American Association for Cancer Research, Inc.)

mAb ME 20.4 against the NGF receptor.[171] The profile of chromatin protein synthesis in proliferating melanocytes is shown in Figure 31, lane 1. Surprisingly, only one protein was labeled with [³⁵S]methionine ($M_r$ 55,000), compared to the very high uptake of [³⁵S]methionine into the chromatin protein of melanoma cells (Figure 8). This indicates that chromatin proteins (nonhistones) of melanocytes are slowly metabolized. The same gel stained by Coomassie blue revealed several bands (not shown). Low turnover of chromatin proteins and a low protein to DNA ratio are in general characteristic for normal cells. After *Eco*RI digestion, the released DNA-protein complex did not show [³⁵S]methionine labeling (Figure 31, lane 2). However, after immunoprecipitation with mAb ME 20.4, a single 230,000-$M_r$ protein was detected by Coomassie blue staining (Figure 31, lane 3), but not by autoradiography. The results indicate that normal melanocytes express a typical high molecular weight chromatin receptor for NGF, which is also found in melanoma cells. However, the receptor expressed in melanocytes shows low turnover, since it does not incorporate [³⁵S]methionine. The fact that the 230,000-$M_r$ protein is detectable by Coomassie blue staining proves that it is expressed in significant amounts.[171]

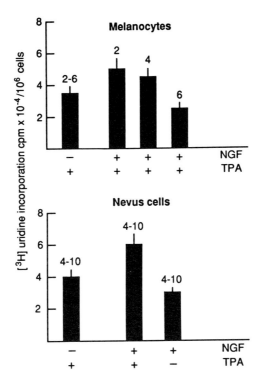

**FIGURE 32.** [³H]uridine incorporation into total intracellular RNA synthesized in melanocytes and in nevus cells incubated for 24 h in the presence or absence of NGF (10 ng/ml). The numbers above the bars indicate the passage number. Data are shown as mean ± SD from three experiments. (From Rakowicz-Szulczynska, E. M., *J. Biol. Reg. Homeostatic Agents,* 6, 21, 1992. With permission of Wichtig Editore.)

## 2. NGF-Regulated Transcription in Melanocytes and Nevus Cells

In order to establish the effect of NGF on RNA synthesis in melanocytes and nevus cells characterized by different ratios of the nuclear to total internalized NGF, the incorporation of [³H]uridine into RNA was tested in cells either exposed or not exposed to NGF.[211]

In melanocytes of the early passages (low n/c NGF ratio), NGF slightly stimulated RNA synthesis (by 10 to 20%). In contrast, in melanocytes of the later passages (high n/c NGF ratio), NGF inhibited RNA synthesis (Figure 32).

In nevus cells growing in the presence of TPA (low n/c NGF ratio), RNA was slightly activated by NGF (Figure 32). When the TPA was removed from the medium, the n/c NGF ratio changed to high, and NGF inhibited RNA synthesis.[211]

The results we obtained suggest that the activatory effect of NGF on RNA synthesis characterizes cells that express a high level of the cell surface receptor and are therefore characterized by a low ratio of n/c NGF. In contrast, in both melanocytes and nevus cells which express a low level of the cell surface receptor and are characterized by a high n/c NGF ratio (Table 12), NGF inhibits RNA synthesis.

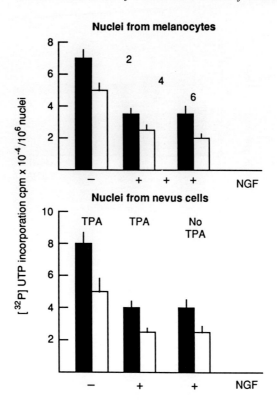

**FIGURE 33.** [³²P]UTP incorporation into total nuclear RNA (dark bar) and rRNA (white bar) synthesized in the isolated nuclei incubated in the presence or absence of NGF (10 ng/ml). Nuclei were isolated from melanocytes growing in the presence of TPA of the passage number indicated above the bars, and from the nevus cells growing either in the presence (+) or absence (−) of TPA. The white bar represents the amount of ³²P-UTP hybridized to the probe of rDNA and therefore represents the level of rRNA synthesis. Data are shown as mean ± SD from three experiments. (From Rakowicz-Szulczynska, E. M., *J. Biol. Reg. Homeostatic Agents,* 6, 21, 1992. With permission of Wichtig Editore.)

To test the function of the chromatin receptor, nuclei isolated from cells of different passages were directly exposed to NGF. In all nuclei, independent of the passage-origin, NGF inhibited incorporation of [³²P]UTP into the synthesized RNA (Figure 33). Hybridization of the synthesized RNA with the probe for the ribosomal DNA indicated that synthesis of ribosomal RNA (Figure 33) in the presence of NGF was 50% lower than in the absence of NGF. The latest results indicated that NGF directly taken up by the nucleus and bound to the chromatin receptor exerts an inhibitory effect on ribosomal DNA synthesis.

Analysis of the results obtained with intact cells (Figure 32) and in a cell-free system (Figure 33) indicates that interaction of NGF with the chromatin receptor always leads to inhibition of rRNA synthesis. Since expression of the chromatin receptor in melanocytes and nevus cells is constant and not modulated by TPA, the effect of NGF on RNA synthesis is the summary effect of the positive regulation,

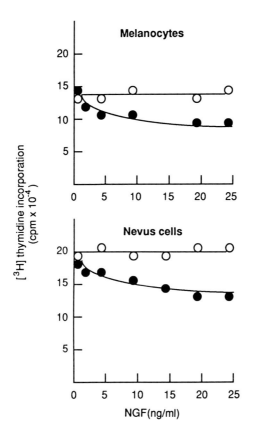

**FIGURE 34.** [³H]thymidine incorporation into DNA of melanocytes (passage 2 ○-○, passage 5 ●-●) and of nevus cells growing in the presence (○-○) or absence (●-●) of TPA. Melanocytes and nevus cells were exposed to NGF for 4 d. (From Rakowicz-Szulczynska, E. M., *J. Biol. Reg. Homeostatic Agents,* 6, 21, 1992. With permission of Wichtig Editore.)

mediated by the cell surface receptor, and of the negative regulation mediated by the chromatin receptor.

## 3. Effect of NGF on Growth of Melanocytes and Nevus Cells

NGF added to the cell culture medium was without any effect on proliferation of melanocytes in early passages or on nevus cells growing in the presence of TPA (Figure 34). However, in later passages of melanocytes and in nevus cells growing in the absence of TPA (high n/c NGF ratio), NGF significantly inhibited growth, as measured by the decreased [³H]thymidine uptake into DNA (Figure 34) and decreased cell number (not shown). The rational interpretation of the results leads to the conclusion that in melanocytes and nevus cells characterized by high nuclear vs. total NGF accumulation (low expression of the cell surface NGF receptor), NGF inhibits growth.[211] We believe that the mechanism of cell growth inhibition by NGF involves the suppressive effect of the NGF-activated chromatin receptor

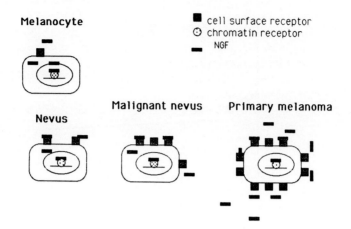

**FIGURE 35.**  Theoretical models of NGF interaction with the cell surface and the chromatin receptors during the melanocyte/nevus cell malignant transformation, leading to primary melanoma. Melanocytes express an extremely low level of cell surface receptors for NGF. NGF does not affect growth of melanocytes, since any stimulatory action of the cell surface receptor is compensated for by the inhibitory effect mediated by the nuclear (chromatin) receptor. Melanocytes express the 230,000-$M_r$ chromatin receptor which shows very low turnover. Nevus cells express more of cell surface receptor for NGF, but the chromatin receptor in those cells is still able to compensate for the effect of the cell surface receptor. Malignant nevus cells express higher levels of NGF cell-surface receptors than melanocytes or non-malignant nevus cells; therefore, the chromatin receptor is no longer able to compensate for the stimulatory effect of the cell surface receptor, and the nevus cells may be stimulated to growth by NGF. Primary melanoma cells exhibit relatively high expression of the cell surface receptor compared to a very low level of the nuclear receptor, and are stimulated to proliferation by NGF. Alternatively, lack of expression of the chromatin receptor may result in NGF-dependent cell growth.

on rRNA synthesis. This negative effect of the chromatin receptor is in the early passages compensated by the cell surface receptor.

In the previous chapter, we showed that WM164 melanoma cells that do not express the nuclear receptor are activated to proliferation by NGF. However, this stimulatory effect of NGF was inverted (switched) to inhibitory when the chromatin receptor for NGF was induced. Melanocytes and nevus cells that express stable levels of the nuclear receptor are inhibited by NGF or stimulated to growth dependent upon the level of expression of the cell surface receptor. Since enhancement of NGF surface receptor expression correlates with the progression of melanocytic cell malignancies, then melanocytes and nevus cells proliferating in the presence of TPA may represent a convenient model for studying NGF action during the first steps of malignant transformation. We can speculate (see Figure 35) that NGF chromatin receptor expressed by normal skin melanocytes acts as a strong inhibitor of cell proliferation. Since normal skin melanocytes express almost undetectable levels of the NGF cell surface receptor, the inhibitory effect of the chromatin receptor is dominant and cells do not proliferate. In nevus cells, expression of the cell surface receptor is higher than on melanocytes, but still sufficiently low to be compensated by the chromatin receptor. However, during the process of malignancy (see malignant nevus and primary melanoma), an increased number of the NGF cell surface receptor may be no longer compensated by the chromatin receptor, and NGF begins to act as cell growth promoter. Alternatively, lack of expression of the chromatin receptor may also switch the effect of NGF to activatory, even if the cell surface receptor is expressed in very low quantities (also observed in WM164 cell lines). Several metastatic melanomas growing *in vitro* express high levels of the cell surface and the chromatin receptor and respond to NGF by inhibiting growth. Whether a sufficiently high concentration of NGF would inhibit growth of melanoma *in vivo* requires further studies.

## D. SWITCH OF NGF FUNCTION DURING NEURONAL DIFFERENTIATION OF HUMAN EMBRYONAL CARCINOMA CELLS

Human embryonal carcinoma 1NTERA-2cl.D1 represents a pluripotent clone of the TERA-2 cell lines, which, in the presence of the retinoic acids, undergoes differentiation into various cell types, including neurons, cells permissive for the replication of human cytomegalovirus, and other cell types.[269-272] Type differentiated cells express specific cell surface markers and may be distinguished from the stem cells.[271-273] We have used the retinoic acid-induced TERA-2 cells as the model for studies on the role of the cell surface and the chromatin receptor for NGF during normal differentiation.[213]

Neuronal differentiation of human TERA-2 (NT2/D1) stem cells was induced by 0 to 4 d of exposure to $10^{-5}$ M all-trans retinoic acid. [125]I-NGF was added for 24 h to the culture of TERA-2 stem cells, and after 7 and 14 d of cell differentiation in the presence of the retinoic acid, cells were fractionated, and distribution of the internalized [125]I-NGF was measured[213] (Table 16). Undifferentiated TERA-2 stem cells exhibited a low level of [125]I-NGF internalization; only 2100 molecules per cell were found inside the cytoplasm and 320 molecules in the chromatin. Cells stimulated for 7 d with the retinoic acid internalized 16,400 molecules per cell, 5400 of which were localized in the chromatin. Cells stimulated 14 d with retinoic acid internalized 4235 molecules of [125]I-NGF per cell, 1000 of which were bound to the chromatin.

In retinoic acid-induced cells, 75% of chromatin-bound [125]I-NGF remained in the chromatin after 0.35 M and 2 M NaCl extraction, which suggests that [125]I-NGF was tightly and specifically bound to the chromatin (Table 15). In TERA-2 stem cells, salt-extracted chromatin contained only 20 molecules of [125]I-NGF, which indicated that chromatin of TERA-2 stem cells did not bind [125]I-NGF specifically. Incubation of cells with [125]I-NGF in the presence of a 100-fold excess of unlabeled NGF blocked incorporation of [125]I-NGF by 90%, which confirmed the specificity of [125]I-NGF uptake (Table 16). The kinetics of [125]I-NGF internalization and the profile of distribution inside undifferentiated and TERA-2 cells stimulated to neuronal differentiation clearly indicate that differentiation is somehow associated with increased expression of the cell surface receptor and with redistribution of NGF from the cytoplasm to the nucleus. Nuclear vs. total accumulation of NGF during

**TABLE 16**

**Intracellular Localization of $^{125}$I-NGF after 24 h Incubation
of TERA-2 Stem Cells and Cells
Exposed 7 or 14 Days to Retinoic Acid**

| Days of incubation with retinoic acid | Cell fraction | $^{125}$I-NGF molecules/cell[a] | |
|---|---|---|---|
| | | A | B |
| 0 | C | 2,500 ± 200 | 290 ± 40 |
| | N | 120 ± 20 | 20 ± 5 |
| | NM | 15 ± 5 | 5 ± 2 |
| | Ch | 400 ± 100 | 50 ± 10 |
| | Ch—0.35 *M*, —2 *M*[b] | 20 ± 10 | 40 ± 8 |
| 2 | C | 5,000 ± 890 | 450 ± 100 |
| | N | 100 ± 20 | 20 ± 5 |
| | NM | 20 ± 5 | 2 ± 1 |
| | Ch | 1,700 ± 250 | 350 ± 50 |
| | Ch—0.35 *M*, —2 *M* | | |
| 7 | C | 12,800 ± 1,500 | 900 ± 100 |
| | N | 550 ± 50 | 300 ± 50 |
| | NM | 150 ± 40 | 20 ± 5 |
| | Ch | 6,000 ± 500 | 700 ± 100 |
| | Ch—0.35 *M*, —2 *M* | 4,200 ± 450 | 300 ± 60 |
| 14 | C | 3,100 ± 500 | 390 ± 40 |
| | N | 80 ± 20 | 20 ± 5 |
| | NM | 10 ± 32 | 5 ± 2 |
| | Ch | 1,200 ± 200 | 300 ± 80 |
| | Ch—0.35 *M*, —2 *M* | 760 ± 120 | 150 ± 50 |

[a]   Number of $^{125}$I-NGF molecules incorporated per cell fraction after 24 h incubation with $^{125}$I-NGF (10 ng/ml) (**A**) or $^{125}$I-NGF (10 ng/ml) plus unlabeled NGF (500 ng/ml) (**B**). Mean ± SD from three experiments.

[b]   The number of $^{125}$I-NGF molecules bound to the chromatin (Ch) after extraction with 0.35 *M* and 2 *M* NaCl.

particular days of differentiation was also tested by indirect immunofluorescence staining of cells exposed to retinoic acids[213] (Figure 36).

Undifferentiated TERA-2 (NT2/D1) cells and cells stimulated 1 to 14 d with the retinoic acid were incubated for 24 h at 37°C with NGF, followed by incubation with rabbit anti-NGF serum and fluoresceine-conjugated goat anti-rabbit IgG (Figure 36). Stem cells showed weak fluorescence of the cytoplasm (Figure 36, day 0). After 1 d of stimulation with retinoic acid, intracellular fluorescence was significantly stronger, and after 2 d, fluorescence of the nucleus was slightly visible. After 4 d of differentiation, fluorescence of the nucleus was stronger than of the cytoplasm, becoming very strong after 7 d of stimulation with retinoic acid. On the next day (day 8), fluorescence of the nucleus began lowering progressively, and after days 12 and 14 fluorescence of the nucleus was very weak and detectable in only 25% of cells. In control experiments, cells were incubated in a NGF-free medium,

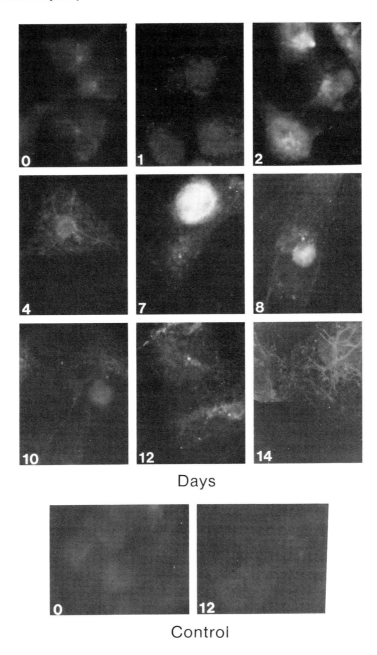

**FIGURE 36.** Immunofluorescence detection of NGF internalized by undifferentiated TERA-2 stem cells (day 0) and TERA-2 cells stimulated with retinoic acid to neuronal differentiation (days 1 to 14). Cells were incubated for 24 h with NGF (10 ng/ml), followed by incubation with anti-NGF rabbit serum and fluoresceine-conjugated goat anti-rabbit IgG. In control experiments, cells were not exposed to NGF.

## TABLE 17
### Effect of NGF (24 h Incubation) on [³H]uridine Incorporation into Cellular RNA of TERA-2 Stem Cells and Cells Stimulated to Differentiation by Retinoic Acid

| Days of incubation with retinoic acid | NGF | [³H]Uridine incorporation (cpm/10⁶ cells)ᵃ | % Synthesis |
|---|---|---|---|
| 0 | − | 17,500 ± 1,500 | 100 |
|   | + | 25,650 ± 4,000 | 143 |
| 2 | − | 20,000 ± 1,500 | 100 |
|   | + | 15,000 ± 2,000 | 75 |
| 7 | − | 25,000 ± 2,000 | 100 |
|   | + | 6,000 ± 200 | 25 |
| 14 | − | 22,000 ± 1,500 | 100 |
|   | + | 14,900 ± 1,000 | 65 |

ᵃ    Data are given as the mean ± SD from three experiments.

followed by incubation with sheep anti-NGF serum and goat anti-rabbit IgG. The control cells did not show fluorescence staining, which eliminates the possibility of nonspecific attachment of goat or sheep IgG to teratocarcinoma cells (Figure 36, control day 0 and day 12). The results indicate that during the first days of neuronal differentiation of TERA-2 cells, the NGF receptor is expressed predominantly in the nucleus, while in differentiated cells, the NGF receptor is expressed predominantly on the plasma membrane. Internalization and nuclear translocation of NGF were inhibited when the cells were exposed to NGF for 30 min at 0°C. At 0°C, both TERA-2 stem cells and the differentiated cells showed only a cell surface fluorescence (not shown).

## 1. Effect of NGF on RNA Synthesis in Intact Cells and in Isolated Nuclei

NGF stimulated [³H]uridine uptake into RNA of TERA-2 stem cells by 150%. After 2 d of stimulation with retinoic acid, NGF inhibited RNA synthesis to 75%, and further inhibited it to 25 and 65% in cells stimulated to differentiation for 7 or 14 d, respectively (Table 17). This inhibitory effect of NGF on RNA synthesis parallels nuclear accumulation of NGF, which was higher after 7 d than after 2 or 14 d. To determine whether the NGF bound to the chromatin directly affected RNA synthesis, nuclei were isolated from TERA-2 stem cells and from cells stimulated 2, 7, or 14 d with retinoic acid and exposed to NGF in a cell-free system (Table 18). In nuclei isolated from TERA-2 stem cells, RNA synthesis was not affected by NGF.

In nuclei isolated after 2, 7, and 14 d of exposure to retinoic acid, RNA synthesis measured as [³²P]UTP incorporation into RNA was inhibited to 50, 14, and 52%, respectively. Hybridization of RNA synthesized in a cell-free system with the probe

## TABLE 18
### Effect of NGF on [$^{32}$P]UTP Incorporation into Total RNA and Ribosomal RNA in Nuclei Isolated from TERA-2 Stem Cells and Cells Exposed to Retinoic Acid

| Days of incubation with retinoic acid | NGF | [$^3$H]UTP incorporation (cpm/10$^6$ nuclei)[a] | % Synthesis | [$^3$H]UTP hybridization to rDNA (cpm) | % Synthesis |
|---|---|---|---|---|---|
| 0 | − | 48,500 | 100 | 21,500 | 100 |
|   | + | 48,200 | 100 | 21,100 | 100 |
| 2 | − | 50,000 | 100 | 21,000 | 50 |
|   | + | 25,000 | 50 | | |
| 7 | − | 55,000 | 100 | 22,000 | 100 |
|   | + | 7,800 | 14 | 500 | 14 |
| 14 | − | 54,000 | 100 | 21,300 | 100 |
|   | + | 27,800 | 52 | 11,000 | 48 |

[a] Data are means from three experiments, SD = 12 to 18%.

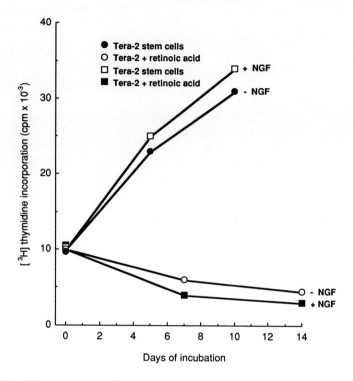

**FIGURE 37.** Effect of NGF on [³H]thymidine incorporation into DNA in TERA-2 stem cells and TERA-2 cells stimulated to neuronal differentiation with retinoic acid.

for rDNA indicated that NGF inhibited rRNA synthesis to 50% after 2 d, to 14% after 7 d, and to 48% after 14 d of differentiation, but was without any effect on rRNA synthesis in nuclei from stem cells. The results suggest that when NGF bound to the chromatin of TERA-2 cells induced to differentiation, rRNA synthesis was inhibited. Since in TERA-2 stem cells NGF did not bind to the chromatin, it did not affect rRNA synthesis. The stimulatory effect of NGF on RNA synthesis in intact cells must be mediated by the cell surface receptor.[213]

## 2. Effect of NGF on Cell Proliferation

TERA-2 stem cells were exponentially growing in cell culture, as indicated by a high uptake of [³H]thymidine into DNA (Figure 37). In the presence of NGF (10 ng/ml), uptake of [³H]thymidine was 15 to 20% higher than in the absence of NGF. Retinoic acid, which induces differentiation, inhibited proliferation of TERA-2 cells, as indicated by progressively decreasing uptake of [³H]thymidine (Figure 37). When NGF (10 ng/ml) was added simultaneously with retinoic acid, [³H]thymidine uptake was by 15 to 25% lower than in the presence of retinoic acid alone. The results obtained indicated that NGF stimulated growth of undifferentiated TERA-2 stem cells. In cells undergoing differentiation, NGF enhanced inhibitory effect of retinoic acid on proliferation of these cells.[213]

## 3. Conclusions

Nuclear accumulation of NGF in retinoic acid-induced teratocarcinoma cells correlates with the inhibitory effect of NGF on ribosomal RNA synthesis and cell proliferation. In undifferentiated stem cells, NGF, which is not bound to the chromatin, does not affect rRNA synthesis. Thus, binding of NGF to the chromatin (receptor) represents a crucial mechanism that leads to inhibition of rRNA synthesis. Stimulation of TERA-2 cell differentiation by the retinoic acid results in cell growth inhibition. However, in the presence of retinoic acid plus NGF, [$^3$H]thymidine incorporation was 15 to 25% lower than in the presence of retinoic acid alone. Thus, NGF enhanced the inhibitory effect of retinoic acid on cell proliferation. In teratocarcinoma cells, nuclear accumulation of NGF and the inhibitory effect of NGF on rRNA synthesis were higher after 7 d than after 14 d. It is likely that in differentiated cells (14 d of exposure), rRNA synthesis must be sufficiently high to keep the protein synthesis and cell metabolism at an appropriate level.

NGF is a factor known to have a critical role in neuronal development. Analysis of the cell surface receptors for NGF did not resolve the mechanism of NGF action. It is likely that the nuclear localization of NGF during the neuronal differentiation and the direct effect of NGF on gene regulation levels represent the key to understanding the molecular events that follow the neuronal differentiation.

## E. MODELS OF NGF INTERACTION WITH rDNA

We suggest that NGF bound to cell-surface receptors mediates a stimulatory effect on cell growth, while the chromatin receptor-bound NGF mediates an inhibitory effect. In cells expressing both receptors, an internalized NGF is taken up by the nucleus and interacts with the chromatin receptor according to the general model of eukaryotic gene regulation. The best characterized is the 230,000-$M_r$ chromatin receptor, typical for melanocytes, melanoma, and glioma cells.

We suggest that at least two mechanisms of NGF interaction with the 230,000-$M_r$ nuclear receptor may be considered (Figure 38). The 230,000-$M_r$ chromatin receptor may be localized in the regulatory region of ribosomal DNA.[174] NGF binding to the 78,000 to 90,000-$M_r$ subunit of the receptor dissociates the 150,000-$M_r$ subunit, which results in conformational changes in DNA (Model 1). Polymerase I does not bind DNA, and the transcription of ribosomal DNA is inhibited. In Model 2, we consider the possibility that the 230,000-$M_r$ dimeric receptor joins two regulatory regions of ribosomal DNA. Dissociation of the 150,000-$M_r$ subunit from the 78,000 to 90,000-$M_r$ subunit in the presence of NGF might result in separation of the two control regions, which, in turn, stops polymerase I binding to DNA (Figure 38, Model 2). These models do not eliminate other possibilities, such as that the 230,000-$M_r$ receptor consists of two identical subunits or more than two subunits and that more complicated interactions may occur.[174] The possibility that NGF directly inhibits activity of polymerase I is unlikely, since, in isolated nuclei of WM164 or TrWM164 cells that do not contain the 230,000-$M_r$ receptor, NGF does not exert any effect on transcription of rRNA. We further suggest that in cells that express both receptors inhibition or activation of proliferation by NGF

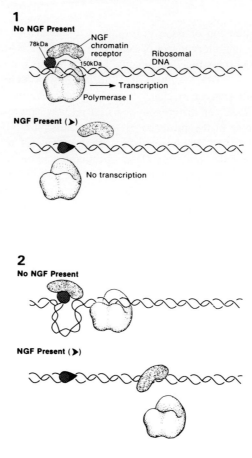

**FIGURE 38.** Hypothetical models of NGF interaction with the chromatin receptor. The 230,000-$M_r$ chromatin receptor for NGF is a nonhistone protein in the regulatory region of ribosomal DNA. In model 1, the oligomeric structure of the receptor is destabilized after binding of NGF. After NGF binds to the 78,000-$M_r$ subunit, the 150,000-$M_r$ subunit dissociates, and the conformational DNA changes do not allow (or they highly reduce) polymerase I interaction with DNA. In Model 2, the 78,000- and 150,000-$M_r$ subunits of the chromatin receptor are both bound to DNA, joining together two regulatory regions of ribosomal DNA. When NGF binds to the 78,000-$M_r$ subunit, the oligomer is destabilized, and the two regulatory regions of DNA separate. Because of the separation, polymerase I binds much less readily to DNA. (From Rakowicz-Szulczynska, E. M., Linnenbach, A., and Koprowski, H., *Mol. Carcinogen.*, 4, 388, copyright © 1991. With permission of Wiley-Liss, division of John Wiley and Sons, Inc.)

may depend on the relative number of chromatin and cell surface receptors. Cells that express a single NGF-binding subunit of the chromatin receptor accumulate NGF in the nucleus, but do not respond to NGF by inhibiting rRNA synthesis. Whether rRNA represents only a nuclear target for NGF or, instead, whether several unique genes are also regulated remains to be investigated. We cannot eliminate a possibility that NGF interacts with nuclear receptors specific for particular cell types and thereby regulates directly different sets of genes. It is likely that alterations of the nuclear receptor structure or function may significantly disturb cell metabolism and lead to uncontrolled growth stimulation.

# V. NUCLEAR RECEPTORS AS THE TARGETS IN CANCER THERAPY

In contrast to the well characterized cell surface receptors for growth factors, the nuclear receptors described by relatively few laboratories represent molecules of existence denied by most established researchers. Analyzing results obtained by particular laboratories (compare Chapters 1 to 3), we have to conclude that there are common points in all these studies; growth factors penetrate the nucleus in a nondegraded form and exhibit very specific localization. Therefore, translocated to the nucleus, growth factors are somehow protected from degradation and bind tightly and specifically to selected chromatin regions. Ribosomal RNA/DNA represent currently the only known targets, common for NGF, FGF, and PDGF. It is noteworthy that both FGF and PDGF are the growth factors that induce the $G_1$ phase of the cell cycle. NGF, which antagonizes the effect of PDGF, acts as an inhibitor of cell division. EGF, IGF-I, or insulin, all of which stimulate progression of the $G_1$ phase, but alone do not induce the $G_1$ phase, do not affect rRNA synthesis. It is likely that in the near future genes regulated by these growth factors would also be discovered.

In most of the models tested thus far, nuclear translocation followed endocytosis of growth factors. We can speculate that at least a fraction of growth factors synthesized by cells may be directly translocated from the cytoplasm to the nucleus. If such an internal loop exists, it would be critical in stimulation of the autocrine growth of cells. In the former case, therapeutics, like mAb or analogs of growth factors, which interact with the cell surface receptors, would be insufficient to block the autocrine mechanism of tumor cell growth, since the active nuclear receptor could regulate cell growth directly on the intracellular level. The new generation of drugs should therefore block not only the cell surface receptors, but the nuclear receptors for growth factors as well. In contrast, drugs which interfere selectively with the cell surface receptors may be either without any effect or may exert partial effect, or even may result in uncontrolled stimulation of the nuclear pathway of the synthesized growth factor.

The presence of the nuclear pathway of external protein-ligands is confirmed by the discovery that some mAb which have been developed against cell surface antigens are able to internalize, enter the nucleus, and bind to the chromatin antigens with an epitopic homology to the cell surface antigens (see Chapters 4 and 5). The last observations further complicate the view of tumor cell growth regulation.

During the past several years, excellent progress has been made in the analysis and cloning of cell surface receptors for growth factors which, however, has not advanced our understanding of cell growth regulation by growth factors and has not clarified the mechanism of tumor cell growth regulation. I hope that the nuclear pathway of growth factors, that unwanted orphan in cancer cell research, will soon not only shed a light on the biology of tumor cells, but will bring new therapeutics acting directly on the DNA level.

## VI. ACKNOWLEDGMENT

I would like to express my gratitude to Mrs. Barbara Piasecka-Johnson and to the J. Seward Johnson Central and East European Study Fund and Paderewski Center, Inc., for sponsoring the major part of these studies.

## REFERENCES

1. **James, J. and Bradshaw, R.,** Polypeptide growth factors, *Annu. Rev. Biochem.,* 53, 259, 1984.
2. **Deuel, T. F.,** Polypeptide growth factors: roles in normal and abnormal cell growth, *Annu. Rev. Cell Biol.,* 3, 443, 1987.
3. **Pimentel, E., Ed.,** *Hormones, Growth Factors, and Oncogenes,* CRC Press, Boca Raton, FL, 1987.
4. **Freeman, C. S., Kimes, B. W., Martin, M. R., and Markes, Ch. L.,** An overview of tumor biology, *Cancer Invest.,* 7, 247, 1989.
5. **Nicolson, G. L.,** Cancer metastasis: tumor cell and host organ properties important in metastasis to specific secondary sites, *Biochim. Biophys. Acta,* 948, 175, 1988.
6. **Rozengurt, E.,** Early signals in the mitogenic response, *Science,* 234, 161, 1986.
7. **Lopez-Rivas, A., Adelberg, E. A., and Rozengurt, E.,** Intracellular $K^+$ and the mitogenic response of 3T3 cells to peptide factors in serum-free medium, *Proc. Natl. Acad. Sci. U.S.A.,* 79, 6275, 1982.
8. **Burns, C. P. and Rozengurt, E.,** Extracellular $Na^+$ and initiation of DNA synthesis: role of intracellular pH and $K^+$, *J. Cell Biol.,* 180, 1082, 1984.
9. **Mendoza, S. A., Lopez-Rivas, A., Sinnett-Smith, J. W., and Rozengurt, E.,** Phorbol esters and diacylglycerol inhibit vasopressin-induced increases in cytoplasmic-free $Ca^{2+}$ and $^{45}Ca^{2+}$ efflux in Swiss 3T3 cells, *Exp. Cell Res.,* 164, 536, 1986.
10. **Owen, N. E. and Villereal, M. L.,** Efflux of $^{45}Ca^{2+}$ from human fibroblasts in response to serum or growth factors, *J. Cell. Physiol.,* 117, 23, 1983.
11. **Berridge, M. J. and Irvine, R. F.,** Inositol trisphosphate, a novel second messenger in cellular signal transduction, *Nature,* 312, 315, 1984.
12. **Nishizuka, Y.,** The role of protein kinase C in cell surface signal transduction and tumor promotion, *Nature,* 308, 693, 1984.
13. **Dicher, P. and Rozengurt, E.,** Phorbol ester stimulation of Na influx and Na-K pump activity in Swiss 3T3 cells, *Biochem. Biophys. Res. Commun.,* 100, 433, 1981.
14. **Gottschalk, W. K. and Jarett, L.,** Intracellular mediators of insulin action, *Diabetes/Metab. Rev.,* 1, 229, 1985.
15. **Gottschalk, W. K., Macaulay, S. L., Macaluary, J. O., Kelly, K., Smith, J. A., and Jarett, L.,** Characterization of mediators of insulin action, *Ann. N.Y. Acad. Sci.,* 488, 385, 1986.
16. **Rozengurt, E., Stroobant, P., Waterfield, M., Deuel, T. F., and Keeham, M.,** Platelet-derived growth factor elicits cyclic AMP accumulation in Swiss 3T3 cells: role of prostaglandin production, *Cell,* 34, 265, 1983.

17. **Coughlin, S. R., Maskowitz, M. A., Zetter, B. R., Antoniades, M. N., and Levine, L.,** Platelet-dependent stimulation of prostacyclin synthesis by platelet-derived growth factor, *Nature,* 288, 600, 1980.

18. **Hunter, T. and Cooper, J. A.,** Protein-tyrosine kinases, *Annu. Rev. Biochem.,* 54, 897, 1985.

19. **Gilman, A. G.,** G proteins and dual control of adenylate cyclase, *Cell,* 36, 577, 1984.

20. **King, L. E., Jr., Carpenter, G., and Cohen, S.,** Characterization by electrophoresis of epidermal growth factor stimulated phosphorylation using A-431 membranes, *Biochemistry,* 19, 1524, 1980.

21. **Das, M., Miyakawa, T., Fox, C. F., Pruss, R. M., Aharonov, A., and Herschman, M. R.,** Specific radiolabelling of a cell-surface receptor for epidermal growth factors, *Proc. Natl. Acad. Sci. U.S.A.,* 74, 2790, 1977.

22. **Hunter, T. and Cooper, J. A.,** Epidermal growth factor induces rapid tyrosine phosphorylation of proteins in A431 human tumor cells, *Cell,* 24, 741, 1981.

23. **Ushiro, H. and Cohen, S.,** Identification of phosphotyrosine as a product of epidermal growth factor-activated protein kinase in A431 cell membranes, *J. Biol. Chem.,* 255, 8363, 1980.

24. **Ek, B., Westermark, B., Wasteson, A., and Heldin, C. M.,** Stimulation of tyrosine-specific phosphorylation by platelet-derived growth factor, *Nature,* 295, 419, 1982.

25. **Nishimura, J., Huang, J. S., and Deuel, T. F.,** Platelet-derived growth factor stimulates tyrosine-specific protein kinase activity in Swiss mouse 3T3 cell membranes, *Proc. Natl. Acad. Sci. U.S.A.,* 79, 4303, 1982.

26. **Kasuga, M., Karlsson, F. A., and Kahn, C. R.,** Insulin stimulates the phosphorylation of the 95,000-dalton subunit of its own receptor, *Science,* 215, 185, 1981.

27. **Shia, M. A. and Pilch, P. F.,** The β subunit of the insulin receptor is an insulin-activated protein kinase, *Biochemistry,* 22, 717, 1983.

28. **Rosen, O. M., Merrera, R., Olowe, Y., Petwzzeli, L. M., and Cabb, M.,** Phosphorylation activates the insulin receptor tyrosine protein kinase, *Proc. Natl. Acad. Sci. U.S.A.,* 80, 3237, 1983.

29. **Jacobs, S., Kull, F. C., Earp, M. S., Svoboda, M. E., Van Wyk, J. J., and Cuatracases, P.,** Somatomalin-C stimulates the phosphorylation of the β-subunit of its own receptor, *J. Biol. Chem.,* 258, 9581, 1983.

30. **Rubin, J. B., Shia, M. A., and Pilch, P. F.,** Stimulation of tyrosine-specific phosphorylation *in vitro* by insulin-like growth factor I, *Nature,* 305, 438, 1983.

31. **Ross, A. M., Grob, P., Bothwell, M., Elder, D. E., Ernst, C. S., Marano, N., Ghrist, B. F. D., Stemp, C. C., Herlyn, M., Atkinson, B., and Koprowski, H.,** Characterization of nerve growth factor receptor in neural crest tumors using monoclonal antibodies, *Proc. Natl. Acad. Sci. U.S.A.,* 81, 6681, 1984.

32. **Chao, M. V., Bothwell, M. A., Ross, A. H., Koprowski, H., Lanahan, A., Budi, C. R., and Sehgal, A.,** Gene transfer and molecular cloning of the human NGF receptor, *Science,* 232, 518, 1986.

33. **Johnson, D., Lanahan, A., Buck, C. R., Sehgal, A., Morgan, C., Mercer, E., Bothwell, M., and Chao, M. V.,** Expression and structure of the human NGF receptor, *Cell,* 47, 545, 1986.

34. **Kaplan, D. R., Hempstead, B. L., Martin-Zanca, D., Chao, M. V., and Parada, L. F.,** The trk protooncogene product: a signal transducing receptor for nerve growth factors, *Science,* 252, 554, 1991.

35. **Klein, R., Jing, S., Nandemi, V., O'Rourke, E., and Barbacid, M.,** The trk proto-oncogene encodes a receptor for nerve growth factor, *Cell,* 65, 189–197, 1991.

36. **Nebreda, A. R., Hempstead, B. L., Martin-Zanca, D., Kaplan, D. R., Parada, L. F., and Santos, E.,** Induction by NGF of meiotic maturation of *Xenopus* oocytes expressing the trk protooncogene product, *Science,* 252, 558, 1991.

37. **Hempstead, B. L., Martin-Zanca, D., Kaplan, D. R., Parada, L. K., and Chao, M. V.,** High affinity NGF binding requires coexpression of the trk proto-oncogene and the low-affinity NGF receptor, *Nature,* 350, 678, 1991.

38. **Crouch, M. F.,** Growth for non-induced cell division is paralleled by translocation of Gi alpha to the nucleus, *FASEB J.,* 5, 200, 1991.
39. **Fields, A. P., Tyler, G., Kraft, A. S., and Mary, W. S.,** Role of nuclear protein kinase C in the mitogenic response to platelet-derived growth factor, *Cell Sci.,* 96, 107, 1990.
40. **Persson, H. and Leder, P.,** Nuclear localization and DNA binding properties of a protein expressed by human c-myc oncogene, *Science,* 225, 718, 1984.
41. **Lin, Y. X. and Vilcek, J.,** Tumor necrosis factor and interleukin-1 cause a rapid and transient stimulation of c-fos and c-myc mRNA levels in human fibroblasts, *J. Biol. Chem.,* 262, 11908, 1987.
42. **Armelin, M. A., Armelin, M. C. S., Kelly, K., Stewart, T. Leder, P., Cochran, B. M., and Stiles, C. D.,** Functional role for c-myc in mitogenic response to platelet-derived growth factor, *Nature,* 310, 655, 1984.
43. **Tsuda, T., Kaibuchi, K., West, B., and Takai, Y.,** Involvement of $Ca^{2+}$ in platelet-derived growth factor-induced expression of c-myc oncogene in Swiss 3T3 fibroblasts, *FEBS Lett.,* 187, 43, 1985.
44. **Ralston, R. and Bishop, J. M.,** The product of the proto-oncogene c-src is modified during the cellular response to platelet-derived growth factor, *Proc. Natl. Acad. Sci. U.S.A.,* 82, 7845, 1985.
45. **Curran, T. and Morgan, J. I.,** Superinduction of c-fos by nerve growth factor in the presence of peripherally active benzodiazepines, *Science,* 229, 1265, 1985.
46. **Kruijer, W., Schubert, D., and Verma, I. M.,** Induction of the proto-oncogene fos by nerve growth factor, *Proc. Natl. Acad. Sci. U.S.A.,* 82, 7330, 1985.
47. **Kelly, K., Cochran, B. H., Stiles, C. D., and Leder, P.,** Cell-specific regulation of the c-myc gene by lymphocyte mitogens and platelet-derived factors, *Cell,* 35, 603, 1983.
48. **Persson, H., Hennighausen, L., Taub, R., De Grado, W., and Leder, P.,** Antibodies to human c-myc oncogene product: evidence of an evolutionarily conserved protein induced during cell proliferation, *Science,* 225, 687, 1984.
49. **Makino, R., Hayashi, K., and Sugimura, T.,** c-myc transcript is induced in rat liver at a very early stage of regeneration or by cycloheximide treatment, *Nature,* 310, 697, 1984.
50. **Kelly, K. and Siebenlist, U.,** The role of c-myc in the proliferation of normal and neoplastic cells, *J. Clin. Immunol.,* 5, 65, 1985.
51. **Carpenter, G. and Cohen, S.,** Epidermal growth factor, *Annu. Rev. Biochem.,* 48, 193, 1979.
52. **Cohen, S., Carpenter, G., and King, L. J.,** Epidermal growth factor-receptor-protein kinase interactions: co-purification of receptor and epidermal growth factor-enhanced phosphorylation activity, *J. Biol. Chem.,* 255, 4834, 1980.
53. **Schlessinger, J.,** Allsotenic regulation of the epidermal growth factor receptor kinase, *J. Cell Biol.,* 103, 2067, 1986.
54. **King, A. C. and Cuatrecasas, P. J.,** Resolution of high and low affinity epidermal growth factor receptors: inhibition of high affinity component by low temperature, cycloheximide and phorbol estres, *J. Biol. Chem.,* 257, 3053, 1982.
55. **Collins, M. J., Sinnett-Smith, J. W., and Rozengurt, E. J.,** Platelet-derived growth factor treatment decreases the affinity of the epidermal growth factor receptors of Swiss 3T3 cells, *J. Biol. Chem.,* 258, 11689, 1983.
56. **Maratos-Flier, E., Yangkao, Ch. Y., Verdin, E. M., and King, G. L.,** Receptor-mediated vectorial transcytosis of epidermal growth factor by madin-derby canine kidney cells, *J. Cell. Biol.,* 105, 1595, 1987.
57. **Gladhaug, I. P. and Christoffersen, T.,** Rapid constitutive internalization and externalization of epidermal growth factor receptors in isolated rat hepatocytes, *J. Biol. Chem.,* 263, 12199, 1988.
58. **Futler, C. E. and Hopkins, C. R.,** Subfractionation of the endocytic pathway: isolation of compartments involved in the processing of internalized epidermal growth factor-receptor complexes, *J. Cell Sci.,* 94, 685, 1989.

59. **Helin, K. and Berguinat, L.**, Internalization and down-regulation of the human epidermal growth factor receptor are regulated by the carboxyl-terminal tyrosines, *J. Biol. Chem.*, 266, 8363, 1991.

60. **Hunter, T., Ling, N., and Cooper, J. A.**, Protein kinase C phosphorylation of the EGR receptor of a threonine residue close to the cytoplasmic face of the plasma membrane, *Nature*, 311, 480, 1984.

61. **Whiteley, B. and Glaser, L. J.**, EGF promotes phosphorylation of threonine-654 of the EGF receptor: possible role of protein kinase C in homogous regulation of the EGF receptor, *J. Cell. Biol.*, 103, 1355, 1986.

62. **Hunter, T. and Cooper, J. A.**, Epidermal growth factor induces rapid tyrosine phosphorylation of proteins in A431 human tumor cells, *Cell*, 24, 741, 1981.

63. **Fava, R. A. and Cohen, S.**, Isolation of a calcium-dependent 35-kilodalton substrate for the epidermal growth factor receptor/kinase from A431 cells, *J. Biol. Chem.*, 259, 2636, 1984.

64. **Novak-Mafer, I. and Thomas, G.**, An activated S6 kinase in extracts from serum- and epidermal growth factor-stimulated Swiss 3T3 cells, *J. Biol. Chem.*, 259, 5995, 1984.

65. **Thomas, G., Martin-Perez, J., Siegmann, M., and Otta, A. M.**, The effect of serum, EGF, $PGF_{2\alpha}$ and insulin on S6 phosphorylation and the initiation of protein and DNA synthesis, *Cell*, 30, 235, 1982.

66. **Lirnch, E., Reiss, N., Berent, E., Ullrich, A., and Schlessinger, J.**, An insertional mutant of epidermal growth factor receptors allows dissection of diverse receptor functions, *EMBO J.*, 6, 2669, 1987.

67. **Honegger, A. M., Szarary, D., Schmidt, A., Lyall, R., Van Obberghen, E., Dull, T. J., Ullrich, A., and Schlessinger, J.**, A mutant epidermal growth factor receptor with defective protein tyrosine kinase is unable to stimulate protooncogene expression and DNA synthesis, *Mol. Cell. Biol.*, 7, 4568, 1987.

68. **Defize, L. H. K., Moolenear, W. H., Van der Saag, P. T., and de Laat, S. W.**, Dissociation of cellular responses to epidermal growth factor using anti-receptor monoclonal antibodies, *EMBO J.*, 5, 1187, 1986.

69. **Gladhaug, I. P. and Christoffersen, T.**, Rapid constitutive internalization and externalization of epidermal growth factor receptors in isolated rat hepatocytes, *J. Biol. Chem.*, 263, 12199, 1988.

70. **Downward, J., Yarden, Y., Mayes, E., Scrace, G., Toffy, N., Stockwell, P., Ullrich, A., Schlessinger, J., and Watrefield, M. D.**, Close similarity of epidermal growth factor receptor and v-erb-b oncogene protein sequences, *Nature*, 307, 521, 1984.

71. **Kondo, I. and Shimizu, N.**, Mapping of the human gene for epidermal growth factor receptor (EGFR) in the p13-q22 region of chromosome 7, *Cytogenet. Cell Genet.*, 35, 9, 1983.

72. **Spurr, N. K., Solomon, E., Jansson, M., Sheer, D., Goodfellow, P. N., Bodmer, W. F., and Vennstrom, G.**, Chromosomal localization of the human homologues to the oncogenes erb A and erb B, *EMBO J.*, 3, 159, 1984.

73. **Graf, T. and Stehelin, D.**, Avian leukemia viruses: oncogenes and genome structure, *Biochem. Biophys. Acta*, 651, 245, 1982.

74. **King, C. R., Kraus, M. H., and Aaronson, S. A.**, Amplification of a novel v-erb B-related gene in a human mammary carcinoma, *Science*, 229, 974, 1985.

75. **Kokai, Y., Dobashi, K., Weiner, D. B., Myers, J. N., Nowell, P. C., and Greene, M. I.**, Phosphorylation process induced by epidermal growth factor alters the oncogenic and cellular neu (NGL) gene products, *Proc. Natl. Acad. Sci. U.S.A.*, 85, 5389, 1988.

76. **Kokai, Y., Meyers, J. N., Wada, T., Brown, V. I., LeVea, C. M., Davis, J. G., Dobashi, K., and Greene, M. I.**, Synergistic interaction of p185-c-neu and the EGF receptor leads to transformation of rodent fibroblasts, *Cell*, 58, 287, 1989.

77. **Kraus, M. H., Popescu, N. C., Amsbaugh, S. C., and King, R. C.**, Expression of the EGF receptor-related protooncogen erb B-2 in human mammary tumor cell lines by different molecular mechanisms, *EMBO J.*, 6, 605, 1987.

78. **Peles, E., Bacus, S. S., Koski, R. A., Lu, H. S., Wen, D., Ogden, S. G., Ben Levy, R., and Yarden, Y.**, Isolation of the Neu/HER-2 stimulatory ligand: a 44-kD glycoprotein that induces differentiation of mammary tumor cells, *Cell,* 69, 205, 1992.

79. **Slamon, D. J., Godolphin, W., Jones, L. A., Holt, J. A., Wong, S. C., Keith, D. E., Levin, W. J., Stuart, S. G., Udore, J., Ullrich, A., and Press, M. F.**, Studies of the HER-2/neu protooncogene in human breast and ovarian cancer, *Science,* 244, 707, 1989.

80. **Lupu, R., Colomer, R., Kannen, B., and Lippmen, M. E.**, Characterization of a growth factor that binds exclusively to the erb B-2 receptor and induces cellular responses, *Proc. Natl. Acad. Sci. U.S.A.,* 89, 2287, 1992.

81. **Todaro, G. J., Fryling, C., and DeLarco, J. E.**, Transforming growth factors produced by certain human tumor cells: polypeptides that interact with epidermal growth factor receptors, *Proc. Natl. Acad. Sci. U.S.A.,* 77, 5258, 1980.

82. **Marquardt, H., Hunkapiller, M. W., Hood, L. E., and Todaro, G. J.**, Rat transforming growth factor type I: structure and relation to epidermal growth factor, *Science,* 223, 1079, 1984.

83. **Reynolds, F. H., Jr., Todaro, G. J., Fryling, C., and Stephenson, J. R.**, Human transforming growth factors induce tyrosine phosphorylation of EGF receptors, *Nature,* 292, 259, 1981.

84. **Pike, L. J., Marquardt, H., Todaro, G. J., Gallis, B., Casnellie, J. E., Bornstein, P., and Krebs, E. G.**, Transforming growth factor and epidermal growth factor stimulate the phosphorylation of a synthetic, tyrosine-containing peptide in a similar manner, *J. Biol. Chem.,* 257, 14628, 1982.

85. **Sainsbury, J. R. C., Farndon, J. R., Sherbet, G. V., and Harris, A. L.**, Epidermal growth factor receptors and estrogen receptors in human breast cancer, *Lancet,* 1, 364, 1985.

86. **Fitzpatrick, S. L., LaChance, M. P., and Schultz, G. S.**, Characterization of epidermal growth factor receptor and action on human breast cancer cells in culture, *Cancer Res.,* 44, 3442, 1984.

87. **Sainsbury, J. R. C., Farndon, J. R., Sherbet, G. V., and Harris, A. L.**, Epidermal growth factor receptors and estrogen receptors in human breast cancer, *Lancet,* i, 364, 1985.

88. **Fitzpatrick, S. L., Brightwell, J., Wittliff, J. L., Barows, G. H., and Schultz, G. S.**, Epidermal growth factor binding by breast tumor biopsies and relationship to estrogen receptor and progestin receptor levels, *Cancer Res.,* 44, 3448, 1984.

89. **Neal, D. E., Marsh, C., Bennett, M. K., Abel, P. D., Mell, R. R., Sainsbury, J. R. C., and Harris, A. L.**, Epidermal growth factor receptors in human bladder cancer: comparisons of invasive and superficial tumors, *Lancet,* 1, 366, 1985.

90. **Basu, M., Murthy, U., Rodeck, U., Herlyn, M., Mattes, L., and Das, M.**, Presence of tumor-associated antigens in epidermal growth factor receptors from different human carcinomas, *Cancer Res.,* 47, 2531, 1987.

91. **Westphal, M., Harsh, G. R., IV, Rosenblum, M. L., and Hammonds, R. G., Jr.**, Epidermal growth factor receptors in the human glioblastoma cell line SF268 differ from those in epidermoid carcinoma cell line A431, *Biochem, Biophys. Res. Commun.,* 132, 284, 1985.

92. **Hendler, F. J. and Ozanne, B. W.**, Human squamous cell lung cancers express increased epidermal growth factor receptors, *J. Clin. Invest.,* 74, 647, 1984.

93. **Koprowski, H., Herlyn, M., Balaban, G., Parmiter, A., Ross, A., and Nowell, P.**, Expression of the receptor for epidermal growth factor correlates with increased dosage of chromosome 7 in malignant melanoma, *Somatic Cell Mol. Genet.,* 11, 297, 1985.

94. **Libermann, J. A., Nusbaum, H. R., Razon, N., Kris, R., Lax, I., Soreq, H., Whittle, N., Waterfield, M. D., Ullrich, A., and Schlessinger, J.**, Amplification, enhanced expression, and possible rearrangement of EGF receptor gene in primary human brain tumors of glial origin, *Nature,* 313, 144, 1985.

95. **Carpenter, G., Stoscheck, C. M., Preston, Y. A., and DeLarco, J. E.**, Antibodies to the epidermal growth factor receptor block the biological activities of sarcoma growth factor, *Proc. Natl. Acad. Sci. U.S.A.,* 80, 5627, 1983.

96. **Hirata, Y., Uchihashi, M., Nakashima, H., Fujita, T., Matsukura, S., and Matsui, K.,** Specific receptors for epidermal growth factor in human bone tumor cells and its effect on synthesis of prostaglandin E by cultured osteosarcoma cell line, *Acta Endocrinol.,* 107, 125, 1984.

97. **Murthy, V., Basu, A., Rodeck, U., Herlyn, M., Ross, A., and Das, M.,** Domain-specificity and antagonistic properties of a new monoclonal antibody to the EGF-receptor, *Arch. Biochem. Biophys.,* 252, 549, 1987.

98. **Rodeck, U., Herlyn, M., Herlyn, D., Molthoff, C., Atkinson, B., Varello, M., Steplewski, Z., and Koprowski, H.,** Tumor growth modulation by a monoclonal antibody to the epidermal growth factor receptor immunologically mediated and effector cell-independent effects, *Cancer Res.,* 47, 3692, 1987.

99. **Brady, L. W., Markoe, A. M., Woo, V. D., Amendola, B. E., Karlsson, U. L., Rackover, M. A., Koprowski, H., Steplewski, Z., and Peyster, R. G.,** Iodine-125-labeled anti-epidermal growth factor receptor-425 in the treatment of glioblastoma multiforme, *Front. Rad. Ther. Oncol.,* 24, 151, 1990.

100. **Brady, L. W., Woo, D. V., Markow, A., Dadparvar, S., Karlsson, U., Rackover, M., Peyster, R., Emrich, J., Miyamoto, C., Steplewski, Z., and Koprowski, H.,** Treatment of malignant gliomas with $^{125}$I-labeled monoclonal antibody against epidermal growth factor receptor, *Antibody Immunoconjugat. Radiopharm.,* 3, 169, 1990.

101. **Epenetos, A. A., Courtenay-Luck, N., Pickering, D., Hooker, G., Durbin, H., Lavender, J. P., and McKenzie, C. G.,** Antibody guided irradiation of brain glioma by arterial infusion of radioactive monoclonal antibody against epidermal growth factor receptor and blood group A antigen, *Br. Med. J.,* 290, 1463, 1985.

102. **Kalofonos, H. P., Pawlikowska, T. R., Hemingway, A., Courtenay-Luck, N., Dhokia, B., Snook, D., Sivolapenko, G. B., Hooker, G. R., McKenzie, C. G., Lavender, P. J., Thomas, D. G. T., and Epenetos, A. A.** Antibody guided diagnosis and therapy of brain gliomas using radiolabeled monoclonal antibodies against epidermal growth factor receptor and placental alkaline phosphatase, *J. Nucl. Med.,* 30, 1636, 1989.

103. **Bender, H., Takahashi, H., Adachi, K., Belser, P., Liang, S., Prewett, M., Schrappe, M., Sutter, A., Rodeck, U., and Herlyn, D.,** Immunotherapy of human glioma xenografts with unlabeled, $^{131}$I- or $^{125}$I-labeled monoclonal antibody 425 to epidermal growth factor receptor, *Cancer Res.,* 52, 121, 1992.

104. **Antoniades, H. N.,** Human platelet-derived growth factor (PDGF): purification of PDGF-I and PDGF-II and separation of their reduced subunits, *Proc. Natl. Acad. Sci. U.S.A.,* 78, 7314, 1981.

105. **Bowen-Pope, D. F. and Ross, R.,** Platelet-derived growth factor, *J. Biol. Chem.,* 257, 5161, 1982.

106. **Glenn, K., Bowen-Pope, D. F., and Ross, R.,** Platelet-derived growth factor, *J. Biol. Chem.,* 257, 5172, 1982.

107. **Deuel, T. F., Huang, J. S., Proffitt, R. T., Baenziger, J. U., Chang, D., and Kennedy, B. B.,** Human platelet-derived growth factor-purification and resolution into two active protein fractions, *J. Biol. Chem.,* 256, 8896, 1981.

108. **Ross, R., Raines, E. W., and Bowen-Pope, D. F.,** The biology of platelet-derived growth factor, *Cell,* 46, 155, 1986.

109. **Heldin, C.-H., Westermark, B., and Wasteson, A.,** Platelet-derived growth factor: isolation by a large-scale procedure and analysis of subunit composition, *Biochem. J.,* 193, 907, 1981a.

110. **Stroobant, P. and Waterfield, M. D.,** Purification and properties of porcine platelet-derived growth factor, *EMBO J.,* 3, 2963, 1984.

111. **Heldin, C.-H., Johnsson, A., Wennergren, S., Wernstedt, C., Betsholtz, C., and Westermark, B.,** A human osteosarcoma cell line secretes a growth factor structurally related to a homodimer of PDGF A-chains, *Nature,* 319, 511, 1986.

112. **Westermark, B., Johnsson, A., Paulsson, Y., Betsholtz, C., Heldin, C.-H., Herlyn, M., Rodeck, U., and Koprowski, H.,** Human melanoma cell lines of primary and metastatic origin express the genes encoding the chains of platelet-derived growth factor (PDGF) and produce a PDGF-like growth factor, *Proc. Natl. Acad. Sci. U.S.A.,* 83, 7197–7200, 1986.

113. **Betsholz, C., Johnsson, A., Heldin, C.-H., Westermark, B., Lind, P., Urdea, M. S., Eddy, R., Shows, T. B., Philpott, K., Mellor, A. L., Knott, T. J., and Scott, J.,** cDNA sequence and chromosomal localization of human platelet-derived growth factor A-chain and its expression in human tumour cells, *Nature,* 320, 695, 1986.

114. **Rakowicz-Szulczynska, E. M. and Koprowski, H.,** Expression of A-type PDGF receptor in cytoplasm of tumor cell lines synthesizing PDGF, *Exp. Mol. Pathol.,* 51, 171, 1989.

115. **Stroobant, P., Gullick, W. J., Waterfield, M. D., and Rozengurt, E.,** Highly purified fibroblast-derived growth factor, an SV40-transformed fibroblast-secreted mitogen, is closely related to platelet-derived growth factor, *EMBO J.,* 4, 1945, 1985.

116. **Waterfield, M. D., Scrace, G. T., Whittle, N., Stroobant, P., Johnsson, A., Wasteson, A., Westermark, B., Heldin, C.-H., Huang, J. S., and Deuel, T. F.,** Platelet-derived growth factor is structurally related to the putative transforming protein p28$^{sis}$ of simian sarcoma virus, *Nature,* 304, 35, 1983.

117. **Devare, S. G., Reddy, E. P., Robbins, K. C., Andersen, P. R., Tronick, S. R., and Aaronson, S. A.,** Nucleotide sequence of the transforming gene of simian sarcoma virus, *Proc. Natl. Acad. Sci. U.S.A.,* 79, 3179, 1982.

118. **Doolittle, R. F., Hunkapiller, M. W., Hood, L. E., Devare, S. G., Robbins, K. C., Aaronson, S. A., and Antoniades, H. N.,** Simian sarcoma virus oncogene, v-*sis*, is derived from the gene (or genes) encoding a platelet-derived growth factor, *Science,* 221, 275, 1983.

119. **Reddy, E. P., Ellmore, N. W., Galen, A. T., Lautenberger, J. A., Papas, T. S., Westin, E. H., Wong-Staal, F., Gallo, R. C., and Aaronson, S. A.,** Cellular genes analogous to retroviral oncogenes are transcribed in human tumor cells, *Nature,* 295, 116, 1982.

120. **Francis, G. E., Michalevicz, R., and Wickremasinghe, R. G.,** Chronic myeloid leukemia and the Philadelphia translocation: do the c-*sis* oncogene and platelet-derived growth factor provide the link?, *Leuk. Res.,* 7, 817, 1983.

121. **Huang, J. S., Huang, S. S., and Deuel, T. F.,** Transforming protein of simian sarcoma virus stimulates autocrine growth of SSV-transformed cells through PDGF cell surface receptors, *Cell,* 39, 79, 1984.

122. **Johnsson, A., Betsholtz, C., von der Helm, K., Heldin, C.-H., and Westermark, B.,** Platelet-derived growth factor against activity of a secreted form of the v-*sis* oncogene product, *Proc. Natl. Acad. Sci. U.S.A.,* 82, 1721, 1985.

123. **Johnsson, A., Heldin, C.-H., Wasteson, A., Westermark, B., Deuel, T. F., Huang, J. S., Seeburg, P. H., Gray, A., Ullrich, A., Scrace, G., Stroobant, P., and Waterfield, M. D.,** The c-*sis* gene encodes a precursor of the B chain of platelet-derived growth factor, *EMBO J.,* 3, 921, 1984.

124. **Josephs, S. F., Dalla Favera, R., Gelmann, E. P., Gallo, R. C., and Wong-Staal, F.,** 5' viral and human cellular sequences corresponding to the transforming gene of simian sarcoma virus, *Science,* 219, 503, 1983.

125. **Josephs, S. F., Guo, C., Ratner, L., and Wong-Staal, F.,** Human proto-oncogene nucleotide sequences corresponding to the transforming region of simian sarcoma virus, *Science,* 223, 487, 1984.

126. **King, C. R., Giese, N. A., Robbins, K. C., and Aaronson, S. A.,** *In vitro* mutagenesis of the v-*sis* transforming gene defines functional domains of its growth factor-related product, *Proc. Natl. Acad. Sci. U.S.A.,* 82, 5295, 1985.

127. **Leal, F., Williams, L. T., Robbins, K. C., and Aaronson, S. A.,** Evidence that the v-*sis* gene product transforms by interaction with the receptor for platelet-derived growth factor, *Science,* 230, 327, 1985.

128. **Deuel, T. F. and Huang, J. S.,** Roles of growth factor activities in oncogenesis, *Blood,* 64, 951, 1984.

129. **Clarke, M. F., Westin, E., Schmidt, D., Josephs, S. F., Ratner, L., Wong-Staal, F., Gallo, R. C., and Reitz, M. S.,** Transformation of NIH 3T3 cells by a human c-*sis* cDNA clone, *Nature*, 398, 464, 1984.

130. **Goustin, A. S., Betsholtz, C., Pfeiffer-Ohlsson, S., Persson, H., Rydnert, J., Bywater, M., Holmgren, G., Heldin, C.-H., Westermark, B., and Ohlsson, R.,** Co-expression of the sis and myc proto-oncogenes in developing human placenta suggests autocrine control of trophoblast growth, *Cell*, 41, 301, 1985.

131. **Heldin, C.-H., Betsholz C., Claesson-Welsh, L., and Westermark, B.,** Subversion of growth regulatory pathways in malignant transformation, *Biochim. Biophys. Acta*, 907, 219, 1987.

132. **Leof, E. B., Proper, J. A., Goustin, A. S., Shipley, G. D., DiCorleto, P. E., and Moses, H. L.,** Induction of c-*sis* mRNA and activity similar to platelet-derived growth factor by transforming growth factor β: a proposed model for indirect mitogenesis involving autocrine activity, *Proc. Natl. Acad. Sci. U.S.A.*, 83, 2453, 1986.

133. **Hermansson, M., Nister, M., Betsholtz, C., Heldin, C.-H., Westermark, B., and Funa, K.,** Endothelial cell proliferation in human malignant glioma: coexpression of mRNA for PDGF B chain and PDGF receptor suggests an autocrine stimulation, *Proc. Natl. Acad. Sci. U.S.A.*, 85, 7748, 1988.

134. **Paulsson, Y., Hammacher, A., Heldin, C.-H., and Westermark, B.,** Possible autocrine feedback in the prereplicative phase of human fibroblasts, *Nature*, 328, 715, 1986.

135. **Betsholtz, C., Westermark, B., Ek, B., and Heldin, C.-H.,** Coexpression of a PDGF-like growth factor and PDGF receptors in a human osteosarcoma cell line: implications for autocrine receptor activation, *Cell*, 39, 447, 1984.

136. **Bywater, M., Rorsman, F., Bongcam-Rudloff, E., Mark, G., Hammacher, A., Heldin, C.-H., Westermark, B., and Betscholtz, C.,** Expression of recombinant platelet-derived growth factor A- and B-chain homodimers in rat-1 cells and human fibroblasts reveals differences in protein processing and autocrine effects, *Mol. Cell Biol.*, 8, 2753, 1988.

137. **Beckmann, M. P., Betsholtz, C., Heldin, C.-H., Westermark, B., Di Fiore, P. P., Robbins, K. C., and Aaronson, S. A.,** Comparison of biological properties and transforming potential of human PDGF-A and PDGF-B chains, *Science*, 241, 1346, 1988.

138. **Grotendorst, G. R., Chang, T., Seppa, H. E. J., Kleinman, H. K., and Martin, G. R.,** Platelet-derived growth factor is a chemoattractant for vascular smooth muscle cells, *J. Cell. Physiol.*, 113, 261, 1982.

139. **Williams, L. T., Antoniades, H. N., and Goetzl, E. J.,** Platelet-derived growth factor stimulates mouse 3T3 cell mitogenesis and leukocyte chemotaxis through different structural determinants, *J. Clin. Invest.*, 72, 1759, 1983.

140. **Heldin, C.-H., Westermark, B., and Wasteson, A.,** Specific receptors for platelet-derived growth factor on cells derived from connective tissue and glia, *Proc. Natl. Acad. Sci. U.S.A.*, 78, 3664, 1981.

141. **Westermark, B., Heldin, C.-H., Ek, B., Johnsson, A., Mellstrom, K., Nister, M., and Wasteson, A.,** Biochemistry and biology of platelet-derived growth factor, in *Growth and Maturation Factors*, Guroff, G., Ed., John Wiley & Sons, New York, 1983, 73.

142. **Ek, B., Westermark, B., Wasteson, A., and Heldin, C.-H.,** Stimulation of tyrosine-specific phosphorylation by platelet-derived growth factor, *Nature*, 295, 419, 1982.

143. **Heldin, C.-H., Bäckström, G., Östman, A., Hammacher, A., Rönnstrand, L., Rubin, K., Nistér, M., and Westermark, B.,** Binding of different dimeric forms of PDGF to human fibroblasts: evidence for two separate receptor types, *EMBO J.*, 7, 1387, 1988.

144. **Matsui, T., Heidaran, M., Miki, T., Popescu, N., La Rochelle, W., Kraus, M., Pierce, J., and Aaronson, S.,** Isolation of a novel receptor cDNA establishes the existence of two PDGF receptor genes, *Science*, 243, 800, 1988.

145. **Berridge, M. Y., Heslop, J. P., Irvine, R. F., and Brown, K. D.,** Inosild trisphosphate formation and calcium mobilization in Swiss 3T3 cells in response to platelet-derived growth factor, *Biochem. J.*, 222, 195, 1984.

146. **Chu, S. M. W., Hoban, C. J., Owen, A. J., and Geyer, R. P.,** Platelet-derived growth factor stimulates polyphosphoinositide breakdown in fetal human fibroblasts, *J. Cell. Physiol.,* 124, 391, 1985.

147. **Coughlin, S. R., Lee, W. M. F., Williams, P. W., Giels, G. M., and Williams, L. T.,** c-myc gene expression is stimulated by agents that activate protein kinase C and does not account for the mitogenic effect of PDGF, *Cell,* 43, 243, 1985.

148. **Assoian, R. K., Grotenolorst, G. R., Miller, D. M., and Sporn, B.,** Cellular transformation by coordinated action of three peptide growth factors from human platelets, *Nature,* 309, 804, 1984.

149. **Huang, J. S., Huang, S. S., and Deuel, T. F.,** Transforming protein of simian sarcoma virus stimulates autocrine cell growth of SSV-transformed cells through PDGF cell-surface receptors, *Cell,* 39, 79, 1984.

150. **Keating, M. T. and Williams, L. T.,** Autocrine stimulation of intracellular PDGF receptors in v-sis in transformed cells, *Science,* 239, 914, 1988.

151. **Johnsson, A., Betsholtz, Ch., Heldin, C.-H., and Westermark, B.,** Antibodies against platelet-derived growth factor inhibit acute transformation by simian sarcoma virus, *Nature,* 317, 438, 1985.

152. **Levi-Montalcini, R.,** Developmental neurobiology and the natural history of nerve growth factor, *Annu. Rev. Neurosci.,* 5, 341, 1982.

153. **Levi-Montalcini, R.,** The nerve growth factor 35 years later, *Science,* 235, 1154, 1987.

154. **Anderson, D. J.,** The neural crest cell lineage problem: neuropoiesis?, *Neuron,* 3, 1, 1989.

155. **Barde, Y. A.,** Trophic factors and neuron survival, *Neuron,* 2, 1525, 1989.

156. **Bothwell, M.,** Keeping track of neurotrophin receptors, *Cell,* 65, 915, 1991.

157. **Chun, L. L. Y. and Patterson, P. M.,** Role of nerve growth factors in the development of rat sympathetic neurons *in vitro.* I. Survival, growth, and differentiation of catecholamine production, *J. Cell Biol.,* 75, 694, 1977.

158. **Raivich, G., Zimmermann, A., and Sutter, A.,** The spatial and temporal pattern of βNGF receptor expression in the developing chick embryo, *EMBO J.,* 4, 637, 1985.

159. **Marushige, Y., Raju, N. R., Marushige, K., and Koestner, A.,** Modulation of growth and of morphological characteristics in glioma cells by nerve growth factor and glia maturation factor, *Cancer Res.,* 47, 4109, 1987.

160. **Apfel, S. C., Lipton, R. B., Arezzo, J. C., and Kessler, J. A.,** Nerve growth factor prevents toxic neuropathy in mice, *Ann. Neurol.,* 29, 87, 1991.

161. **Scarpini, E., Ross, A. H., Rosen, J. L., Brown, M. J., Rostami, A., Koprowski, H., and Lisak, R. P.,** Expression of nerve growth factor receptor during human peripheral nerve development, *Dev. Biol.,* 125, 301, 1988.

162. **Davies, A. M., Bandtlow, C., Heumann, R., Korsching, S., Rohrer, H., and Thoenen, N.,** Timing site of nerve growth factor synthesis in developing skin in relation to innervation and expression of the receptor, *Nature,* 326, 353, 1987.

163. **Anderson, P. J. and Axel, R.,** A bipotential neuroendocrine precursor, whose choice of cell fate is determined by NGF and glucocorticoids, *Cell,* 47, 1079, 1985.

164. **Lillien, L. E. and Claude, P.,** Nerve growth factor is a mitogen for cultured chromaffin cells, *Nature,* 317, 632, 1985.

165. **Stemple, D. L., Mahanthappa, N. K., and Anderson, D. J.,** Basic FGF induces neuronal differentiation, cell division, and NGF dependence in chromaffin cells: a sequence of events in sympathetic development, *Neuron,* 1, 517, 1988.

166. **Unsicker, K., Krisch, B., Otten, J., and Thoenen, H.,** Nerve growth factor-induced fiber outgrowth from isolated rat adrenal chromaffin cells: impairment by glucocorticoids, *Proc. Natl. Acad. Sci. U.S.A.,* 75, 3498, 1978.

167. **Fabricant, R. N., DeLarco, J. E., and Todaro, G. J.,** Nerve growth factor receptors on human melanoma cells in culture, *Proc. Natl. Acad. Sci. U.S.A.,* 74, 565, 1977.

168. **Grob, P. M., Ross, A. M., Koprowski, H., and Bothwell, M. A.,** Characterization of the human membrane nerve growth factor receptors, *J. Biol. Chem.,* 260, 8044, 1985.

169. **Greene, L. A. and Tischler, A. S.,** PC12 pheochromocytoma cultures in neurobiological research, *Adv. Cell. Neurol.,* 3, 373, 1982.
170. **Rudkin, B. B., Lazarovici, P., Levi, B. Z., Abe, Y., Fujita, K., and Gunoff, G.,** Cell cycle-specific action of nerve growth factor in PC12 cells: differentiation without proliferation, *EMBO J.,* 8, 3319, 1989.
171. **Rakowicz-Szulczynska, E. M., Herlyn, M., and Koprowski, H.,** Nerve growth factor receptors in chromatin of melanoma cells, proliferating melanocytes and colorectal cells *in vitro, Cancer Res.,* 48, 7200, 1988.
172. **Rakowicz-Szulczynska, E. M. and Koprowski, H.,** Antagonistic effect of PDGF and NGF on transcription of ribosomal DNA and tumor cell proliferation, *Biochim. Biophys. Res. Commun.,* 163, 649, 1989.
173. **Rakowicz-Szulczynska, E. M., Linnenbach, A., and Koprowski, H.,** Intracellular receptor binding and nuclear transport of nerve growth factor in intact cells and a cell-free system, *Mol. Carcinogen.,* 2, 47, 1989.
174. **Rakowicz-Szulczynska, E. M., Reddy, U., Vorbrodt, A., Herlyn, D., and Koprowski, H.,** Cell surface and the chromatin receptor mediated melanoma cell growth response to NGF, *Mol. Carcinogen.,* 4, 388, 1991.
175. **Rakowicz-Szulczynska, E. M., Rodeck, U., Herlyn, M., and Koprowski, H.,** Chromatin binding of epidermal growth factor, nerve growth factor, and platelet-derived growth factor in cells bearing the appropriate surface receptors, *Proc. Natl. Acad. Sci. U.S.A.,* 83, 3728, 1986.
176. **Rakowicz-Szulczynska, E. M., Mozdzanowski, J., Lundberg, T., Kaczmarski, W., and Speicher, D.,** Gamma-interferon-induced expression of NGF chromatin receptor in colorectal carcinoma cells, *Growth Factors,* 6, 337, 1992.
177. **Radeke, M. J., Misko, T. P., Hsu, Ch., Merzenberg, L. A., and Shooter, E. M.,** Gene transfer and molecular cloning of the rat nerve growth factor receptor, *Nature,* 25, 593, 1987.
178. **Maher, P. A.,** Nerve growth factor-induced protein kinase phosphorylation, *Proc. Natl. Acad. Sci. U.S.A.,* 85, 6788, 1988.
179. **Martin-Zanca, D., Oskam, R., Mitra, G., Copeland, T., and Barbacid, M.,** Molecular and biochemical characterization of the human trk proto-oncogene, *Mol. Cell. Biol.,* 9, 24–33, 1989.
180. **Kaplan, D. A., Martin-Zance, D., and Peraola, Z.,** Tyrosine phosphorylation and tyrosine kinase activity of the trk proto-oncogene product induced by NGF, *Nature,* 350, 158, 1991.
181. **Rodriguez-Tébar, A., Dechant, G., and Barde, Y.-A.,** Binding of brain-derived neurotrophic fiber to the nerve growth factor receptor, *Neuron,* 4, 487, 1990.
182. **Squinto, S. P., Stitt, T. N., Aldrich, T. H., Davis, S., Bianco, S. M., Radziewski, C., Glass, D. J., Masiakowski, P., Furth, M. E., Valenzuela, D. M., DiStefano, P. S., and Yancopoulos, G. D.,** trk B encodes a functional receptor for brain-derived neurotrophic factor and neurotrophin 3 but not nerve growth factor, *Cell,* 65, 885, 1991.
183. **Soppet, D., Escandon, E., Maragos, J., Middlemas, D. S., Reid, S. W., Blair, J., Burton, L. E., Stanton, B. R., Kaplan, D. R., Hunter, T., Nikolics, K., and Parada, L. F.,** The neurotrophic factor-brain-derived neurotrophic factor and neurotrophic-3 are ligands for the trk B tyrosine kinase receptor, *Cell,* 65, 895, 1991.
184. **Lamballe, F., Klein, R., and Barbacid, M.,** trk C, a new member of the trk family of tyrosine protein kinases, is a receptor for neurotrophin-3, *Cell,* 66, 967, 1991.
185. **Thoenen, H., Angeletti, P. U., Levi-Montatcini, R., and Kettler, R.,** Selective induction of tyrosine hydroxylase and dopamine hydroxylase in rat superior cervical ganglia by nerve growth factor, *Proc. Natl. Acad. Sci. U.S.A.,* 68, 1598, 1971.
186. **Greene, L. A. and Rein, G.,** Synthesis, storage, and release of acetylcholine by a nerve-growth factor responsive line of rat pheochromocytoma cells, *Nature,* 268, 349, 1977.
187. **Rieger, F., Shelanski, M. L., and Greene, L. A.,** The effects of nerve growth factor on acetylcholinesterase and its multiple forms in cultures of rat PC12 pheochromocytoma cells: increased total specific activity and appearance of the 16S molecular form, *Dev. Biol.,* 76, 238, 1980.

188. **Liuzzi, A., Foppen, F. H., and Kopin, I. J.,** Stimulation and maintenance by nerve growth factor of phenylethanolamine-N-methyltransferase in superior cervical ganglia of adult rats, *Brain Res.,* 138, 309, 1977.
189. **MacDonnell, P. G., Nagaich, K., Lakshmanan, J., and Guroff, G.,** Nerve growth factor increases activity of ornithine decarboxylase in superior cervical ganglion of young rats, *Proc. Natl. Acad. Sci. U.S.A.,* 74, 4681, 1977.
190. **Feinstein, S. C., Dana, S. L., McConlogue, L., Shooter, E. M., and Coffino, P.,** Nerve growth factor rapidly induces ornithine decarboxylase mRNA in PC12 rat pheochromocytoma cells, *Proc. Natl. Acad. Sci. U.S.A.,* 82, 5761, 1985.
191. **Greene, L. A. and Shooter, E. M.,** The nerve growth factor: biochemistry, synthesis, and mechanism of action, *Annu. Rev. Neurosci.,* 3, 353, 1980.
192. **Chandler, C. E., Cragoe, E. J., Jr., and Glaser, L.,** Nerve growth factor does not activate $Na^+/H^+$ exchange in PC12 pheochromocytoma cells, *J. Cell. Physiol.,* 125, 367, 1985.
193. **Greenberg, M. E., Greene, L. A., and Ziff, E. B.,** Nerve growth factor and epidermal growth factor induce rapid transient changes in proto-oncogene transcription in PC12 cells, *J. Biol. Chem.,* 260, 14101, 1985.
194. **Halegoua, S. and Patrick, J.,** Nerve growth factor mediates phosphorylation of specific proteins, *Cell,* 22, 571, 1980.
195. **Nakanishi, N. and Guroff, G.,** Nerve growth factor-induced increase in the cell-free phosphorylation of a nuclear protein in PC12 cells, *J. Biol. Chem.,* 260, 7791, 1985.
196. **Masiakowski, P. and Shooter, E. M.,** Nerve growth factor induces the genes for two proteins related to a family of calcium-binding proteins in PC12 cells, *Proc. Natl. Acad. Sci. U.S.A.,* 85, 1277, 1988.
197. **Leonard, D. G. B., Gorham, J. D., Cole, P., Greene, L. A., and Ziff, E. B.,** A nerve growth factor-regulated messenger RNA encodes a new intermediate filament protein, *J. Cell Biol.,* 106, 181, 1988.
198. **Brown, M. S., Anderson, A. G. W., and Goldstein, J. L.,** Recycling receptors: the round-tip itinerary of migrant membrane proteins, *Cell,* 32, 663, 1983.
199. **Hanover, J. A., Willinghem, M. C., and Pastan, I.,** Kinetics of transit of transferrin and epidermal growth factor through clathrin-coated membranes, *Cell,* 39, 283, 1984.
200. **Heldin, C. N., Wasteson, A., and Westermark, B.,** Interaction of platelet-derived growth factor with its fibroblast receptor: demonstration of ligand degradation and receptor modulation, *J. Biol. Chem.,* 257, 4216, 1982.
201. **Rosenfeld, M. E., Bowen-Pope, D. F., and Ross, R.,** Platelet-derived growth factor: morphologic and biochemical studies of binding, internalization, and degradation, *J. Cell. Physiol.,* 121, 263, 1984.
202. **Carpenter, G. and Cohen, S.,** $^{125}I$-labeled human epidermal growth factor: binding, internalization, and degradation in human fibroblasts, *J. Cell Biol.,* 71, 159, 1976.
203. **Rohrer, M., Schäfer, T., Korsching, S., and Thoenen, M.,** Internalization of nerve growth factor by pheochromocytome PC12 cells: absence of transfer to the nucleus, *J. Neurosci.,* 2, 687, 1982.
204. **Bikfalvi, A., Dupruy, E., Inyong, A. L., Fayein, N., Leseche, G., Courtois, Y., and Tobelern, G.,** Binding, internalization, and deregulation of basic fibroblast growth factor in human microvascular endothelial cells, *Exp. Cell Res.,* 181, 75, 1989.
205. **Andres, R. Y., Jeng, I., and Bradshaw, R. A.,** Nerve growth factor receptors: identification of distinct classes in plasma membranes and nuclei of embryonic dorsal root neurons, *Proc. Natl. Acad. Sci. U.S.A.,* 77, 2785, 1977.
206. **Yanker, B. A. and Shooter, E. M.,** Nerve growth factor in the nucleus: interaction with receptors on the nuclear membrane, *Proc. Natl. Acad. Sci. U.S.A.,* 76, 1269, 1979.
207. **Marchisio, P. C., Naldini, L., and Calissano, P.,** Intracellular distribution of nerve growth factor in rat pheochromocytoma PC12 cells: evidence for a perinuclear and intranuclear location, *Proc. Natl. Acad. Sci. U.S.A.,* 77, 1656, 1980.

208. **Calissano, P. and Cozzani, C.**, Interaction of nerve growth factor with the mouse-brain neurotubule protein(s), *Proc. Natl. Acad. Sci. U.S.A.*, 71, 2131, 1974.

209. **Piovo, E. P., Ribeiro-da-Silva, A., and Cuello, A. C.**, Immunoelectron microscopic evidence of nerve growth factor receptor metabolism and internalization in rat nucleus basalic neurons, *Brain Res.*, 527, 109, 1990.

210. **Rakowicz-Szulczynska, E. M. and Koprowski, H.**, Identification of NGF receptor in chromatin of melanoma cells, using monoclonal antibody to cell surface receptor, *Biochem. Biochim. Res. Commun.*, 140, 174, 1986.

211. **Rakowicz-Szulczynska, E. M.**, Nerve growth factor chromatin receptor and cell surface receptor-regulated growth of melanocytes and nevus cells, *J. Biol. Reg. Homeostatic Agents*, 6, 21, 1992.

212. **Rakowicz-Szulczynska, E. M.**, Identification of the cell surface and nuclear receptors for NGF in breast carcinoma cell lines, *J. Cell Physiol.*, 154, 64, 1993.

213. **Rakowicz-Szulczynska, E. M.**, unpublished data.

214. **Rakowicz-Szulczynska, E. M.**, unpublished data.

215. **Wetmore, C., Cao, Y., Petterson, R. F., and Olson, L.**, Brain-derived neurotrophic factor: subcellular compartmentalization and interneuronal transfer as visualized with anti-peptide antibodies, *Proc. Natl. Acad. Sci. U.S.A.*, 88, 9843, 1991.

216. **Johnson, L. K., Baxter, J. D., Vlodavsky, I., and Gospodarowicz, D.**, Epidermal growth factor and expression of specific genes: effects on cultured rat pituitary cells are dissociable from the mitogenic response, *Proc. Natl. Acad. Sci. U.S.A.*, 77, 394, 1980.

217. **Johnson, L. K., Vlodavsky, I., Baxter, J. D., and Gospodarowicz, D.**, Nuclear accumulation of epidermal growth factor in cultured rat pituitary cells, *Nature*, 287, 340, 1980.

218. **Savion, N. S., Vlodavsky, I., and Gospodarowicz, D.**, Nuclear accumulation of epidermal growth factor in cultured bovine corneal endothelial and granulosa cells, *Nature*, 256, 1149, 1981.

219. **Murawsky, Y., Storkermaier, R., Fleig, W. E., and Hahn, E. G.**, Effects of chloroguine and hapetic stimulator substance on cellular accumulation and nuclear binding of $^{125}$I-epidermal growth factor in primary culture of adult rat hepatocytes, *Res. Commun. Chem. Pathol. Pharmacol.*, 69, 3, 1990.

220. **Rakowicz-Szulczynska, E. M., Otwiaska, D., Rodeck, U., and Koprowski, H.**, Epidermal growth factor (EGF) and monoclonal antibody to the cell surface EGF receptor bind to the same chromatin receptor, *Arch. Biochem. Biophys.*, 268, 456, 1989.

221. **Rakowicz-Szulczynska, E. M., Steplewski, Z., and Koprowski, H.**, Internalization and nuclear translocation of a monoclonal antibody to a carbohydrate Y determinant, *Am. J. Pathol.*, 141, 937, 1992.

222. **van den Eijnden-van Raaij, A. J. M., van Maurik, P., Boonstra, J., van Zoelen, E. J. J., and de Laat, S. W.**, Ultrastructural localization of platelet-derived growth factor and related factors in normal and transformed cells, *Exp. Cell Res.*, 178, 479, 1988.

223. **Yeh, H.-Y., Pierce, G. F., Pierce, G. F., and Deuel, T. F.**, Ultrastructural localization of a platelet-derived growth factor/v-*sis*-related protein(s) in cytoplasm and nucleus of simian sarcoma virus-transformed cells, *Proc. Natl. Acad. Sci. U.S.A.*, 84, 2327, 1987.

224. **Lee, B. A., Maher, D. W., Mannink, M., and Donoghue, D. J.**, Identification of a signal for nuclear targeting in platelet-derived growth-factor-related molecules, *Mol. Cell. Biol.*, 7, 3527, 1987.

225. **Pierce, G. F., Shawver, L. K., Milner, P. G., Yeh, M. J., Thomason, A., and Deuel, T. S.**, Identification and purification of PDGF/*sis*-like proteins from nuclei of simian sarcoma virus-transformed fibroblasts, *Oncogene Res.*, 2, 235, 1988.

226. **Bouche, G., Gas, N., Prats, M., Baldin, U., Tauber, J. P., Terssie, J., and Amalric, F.**, Basic fibroblast growth factor enters the nucleolus and stimulates the transcription of ribosomal genes in ABAE cells undergoing $G_0 \rightarrow G_1$ transition, *Proc. Natl. Acad. Sci. U.S.A.*, 84, 7660, 1987.

227. **Baldin, V., Roman, A. M., Bosc-Bierne, I., Amalvic, F., and Bouche, G.,** Translocation of bFGF to the nucleus in G₁ phase cell cycle specific in bovine aortic endothelial cells, *EMBO J.,* 9, 1511, 1990.

228. **Tessler, S. and Neufeld, G.,** Basic fibroblast growth factor accumulates in the nuclei of various bFGF-producing cell types, *J. Cell. Physiol.,* 145, 310, 1990.

229. **Lee, N. D. and Williams, R. M.,** *Endocrinology,* 54, 5, 1955.

230. **Arguilla, E. R.,** 67th Annual Meeting of the American Association of Pathology and Bacteriology, St. Louis, MO, March, 1970, 692 (Abstr. No. 134).

231. **Goldfine, I. D., Smith, G. J., Wong, K. Y., and Jones, A. L.,** Cellular uptake and nuclear binding of insulin in human cultured lymphocytes. Evidence for potential intracellular sites of insulin action, *Proc. Natl. Acad. Sci. U.S.A.,* 74, 1368, 1977.

232. **Vigneri, R., Goldfine, I. D., Wong, K. Y., Smith, G. J., and Pezzino, V.,** The nuclear envelope, *J. Biol. Chem.,* 253, 2098, 1978.

233. **Smith, R. M. and Jarett, L.,** Ultrastructural evidence for the accumulation of insulin in the nuclei of intact 3T3-L1 adipocytes by an insulin-receptor mediated process, *Proc. Natl. Acad. Sci. U.S.A.,* 84, 459, 1987.

234. **Podlecki, D. A., Smith, R. M., Kao, M., and Jarett, L.,** Nuclear translocation of the insulin receptor, *J. Biol. Chem.,* 262, 3362, 1987.

235. **Rakowicz-Szulczynska, E. M., Otwiaske, D., and Koprowski, H.,** Plasma membrane-mediated nuclear uptake and chromatin binding of insulin in tumor cell lines, *Mol. Carcinogen.,* 3, 150, 1990.

236. **Soler, A. P., Alemany, J., Smith, R. M., de Pablo, F., and Jarett, L.,** The state of differentiation of embryonic chicken lens cells determines insulin-like growth factor I internalization, *Endocrinology,* 127, 595, 1990.

237. **Falk, W., Von Hogen, I., and Kramer, P. H.,** Activation of T cells by interleukin 1 involves internalization of interleukin 1, *Lymphokine Res.,* 8, 263, 1989.

238. **Grenfell, S., Smithers, N., Miller, K., and Solari, R.,** Receptor-mediated endocytosis and nuclear transport of human interleukin 1 alpha, *J. Biol. Chem.,* 264, 813, 1989.

239. **Re, R. N., MacPhee, A. A., and Fallon, J. F.,** Specific nuclear binding of angiotensin II, *Clin. Sci.,* 61, 2455, 1981.

240. **Re, R. N., LaBiche, R. A., and Bryan, S. E.,** Nuclear-hormone mediated changes in chromatin solubility, *Biochem. Biochim. Res. Commun.,* 110, 61, 1983.

241. **Re, R. N., Vizarol, D. L., Brown, J., and Bryan, S. E.,** Angiotensin II receptors in chromatin fragments generated by micrococcal nuclease, *Biochem. Biochim. Res. Commun.,* 119, 220, 1984.

242. **Re, R. N. and Parob, M.,** Effect of angistensin II or RNA synthesis by isolated nuclei, *Life Sci.,* 34, 647, 1984.

243. **Omary, M. B. and Kagnoft, M. F.,** Identification of nuclear receptors for VIP on a human colonic adenocarcinoma cell line, *Science,* 238, 1578, 1987.

244. **Clevenger, C. V., Sillmen, A. L., and Prystowsky, M. B.,** Interleukin-2 driven nuclear translocation of protection in cloned T lymphocytes, *Endocrinology,* 127, 3151, 1990.

245. **Laemmli, U. K.,** Cleavage of structural proteins during the assembly of the head of bacteriophage T4, *Nature,* 227, 680, 1971.

246. **Rakowicz-Szulczynska, E. M. and Horst, A.,** Non-histone proteins in fractionated chromatin before and after DNaseII treatment, *Biochim. Biophys. Acta,* 69, 653, 1991.

247. **Rakowicz-Szulczynska, E. M. and Horst, A.,** Differences in salt solubility, DNaseII sensitivity and template activity of chromatin from antibody synthesizing spleen cells and myeloma cells RPC5 and ABPC22, *Mol. Cell. Biochem.,* 48, 71, 1982.

248. **O'Farrell, P. M.,** High resolution two-dimensional electrophoresis of proteins, *J. Biol. Chem.,* 250, 4007, 1975.

249. **Rakowicz-Szulczynska, E. M., Linnenbach, A., and Koprowski, H.,** Rapid and sensitive method to detect expression of growth factor receptors, *J. Immunol. Methods,* 3, 150, 1989.

250. **Lengyel, P.,** Biochemistry of interferons and their actions, *Annu. Rev. Biochem.,* 51, 251, 1982.

251. **Sidky, T. A., Borden, E. C., Wierenga, W., and Bryan, G. T.,** Inhibitory effects of interferon-inducing pyrimidinones on the growth of transplantable mouse bladder tumors, *Cancer Res.,* 46, 3798, 1986.

252. **Borden, E., Sidky, T. A., Erturk, E., Wierenga, W., and Bryan, G. T.,** Protection from carcinogen-induced murine bladder carcinoma by interferons and in oral interferon-inducing pyrimidinone, bropirimine, *Cancer Res.,* 50, 1071, 1990.

253. **Borden E. C., Groveman, D. S., Nasu, T., Resnikiff, C. A., and Bryan, G. T.,** Antiproliferative activities of interferons against human bladder carcinoma cell lines *in vitro, J. Urol.,* 132, 800, 1984.

254. **Balkwill, F. and Taylor-Papadimitrow, J.,** Interferon affects both $G_1$ and $StG_2$ in cells stimulated from quiescence to growth, *Nature,* 274, 798, 1978.

255. **Grossberg, S. E. and Keay, S.,** The effects of interferon on 3T3-L1 cell differentiation, *Ann. N.Y. Acad Sci.,* 350, 294, 1980.

256. **Friedman, R. L., Manly, S. P., McMahon, M., Kerr, I. M., and Stark, G. R.,** Transcriptional and posttranscriptional regulation of interferon-induced gene expression in human cells, *Cell,* 38, 745, 1984.

257. **Dale, T., Ali Imam, A. M., Kerr, I. M., and Stark, G. R.,** Rapid activation by interferon $\alpha$ of a latent DNA-binding protein present in the cytoplasm of untreated cells, *Proc. Natl. Acad. Sci. U.S.A.,* 86, 1203, 1989.

258. **Cohen, B., Peretz, B., Vaiman, D., Benech, P., and Chebath, J.,** Enhancer-like interferon responsive sequences of the human and murine ($2' — 5'$) oligoadenylate synthetase gene promoter, *EMBO J.,* 7, 1411, 1988.

259. **Proter, A. C. G., Chernajovsky, Y., Dale, T. C., Gilbert, C. S., Stark, G. R., and Kerr, I. M.,** Interferon response element of the human gene 6-16, *EMBO J.,* 7, 85, 1988.

260. **Tominaga, S. and Tominaga, K.,** Interferon alters the pattern of secreted proteins from Ehrlich ascites-tumor cells, *Biochem. J.,* 261, 57, 1989.

261. **Tominaga, S. and Lengyel, P.,** $\beta$-interferon alters the pattern of proteins secreted from quiescent and platelet-derived growth factor-truncated BA$^1$B/C-3T3 cells, *J. Biol. Chem.,* 260, 1975, 1985.

262. **Stamenkovic, I., Clark, E. A., and Seed, B.,** A B-lymphocyte activation molecule related to the nerve growth factor receptor and introduced by cytokines in carcinomas, *EMBO J.,* 8, 1403, 1989.

263. **Herlyn, M., Rodeck, U., Mancianti, M. L., Cardillo, F. M., Lang, A., Ross, A. H., Jambrosic, J., and Koprowski, H.,** Expression of melanoma-associated antigens in cultured rapidly dividing human melanocytes, *Cancer Res.,* 47, 3057, 1987.

264. **Herlyn, M., Mancianti, M. L., Jambrosic, J., Bolen, J. B., and Koprowski, H.,** Regulatory factors that determine growth and phenotype of normal human melanocytes, *Exp. Cell Res.,* 179, 322, 1988.

265. **Mancianti, M. L., Herlyn, M., Weil, D., Jambrosic, J., Rodeck, U., Becker, D., Diamond, L., Clark, W. H. Jr., and Koprowski, H.,** Growth and phenotypic characteristic of human nevus cells in culture, *J. Invest. Dermatol.,* 90, 134, 1988.

266. **Elder, D. E., Rodeck, U., Thurin, J., Cardillo, F., Clark, W. H., Stewart, R., and Herlyn, M.,** Antigenic profile of tumor progression stages in human melanocytic nevi and melanomas, *Cancer Res.,* 49, 5091, 1989.

267. **Herlyn, M. H., Clark, W. H., Rodeck, U., Mancianti, M. L., Jambrosic, J., and Koprowski, H.,** Biology of disease: biology of tumor progression in human melanocytes, *Lab. Invest.,* 56, 461, 1987.

268. **Bröcker, E. B., Magiera, H., and Herlyn, M.,** Nerve growth and expression of receptors for nerve growth factor in tumors of melanocyte origin, *J. Invest. Dermatol.,* 96, 662, 1991.

269. **Anderson, P. J. and Axel, R.,** A bipotential neuroendocrine precursor whose choice of cell fate is determined by NGF and glucocorticoids, *Cell,* 47, 1079, 1985.

270. **Andrews, P. W., Goodfellow, P. N., Shevinsky, L., Bronson, D. L., and Knowles, B. B.,** Cell surface antigens of a clonal human embryonal carcinoma cell line: morphological and antigenic differentiation in culture, *Int. J. Cancer,* 29, 523, 1982.

271. **Andrews, P. W.**, Retinoic acid induces neuronal differentiation of a cloned human embryonal carcinoma cell line *in vitro, Dev. Biol.*, 103, 285, 1984.

272. **Andrews, P. W., Damjanov, I., Simon, D., Banting, G., Carlin, C., Dracopoli, N. C., and Fogh, J.**, Pluripotent embryonal carcinoma clones derived from the human teratocarcinoma cell lines TERA-2: differentiation *in vivo* and *in vitro, Lab. Invest.*, 50, 147, 1984.

273. **Damjanov, I. and Andrews, P. W.**, Ultrastructural differentiation of a clonal human embryonal carcinoma cell line *in vitro, Cancer Res.*, 43, 2190, 1983.

Chapter 2

# NUCLEAR LOCALIZATION OF ACIDIC AND BASIC FIBROBLAST GROWTH FACTOR (FGF)

G. Bouche, A. M. Roman, I. Truchet, M. Guyader, V. Baldin,
L. Créancier, P. Brethenou, Y. Courtois, and F. Amalric

## TABLE OF CONTENTS

0-8493-4713-0/94/$0.00 + $.50

# I. INTRODUCTION

Acidic and basic fibroblast growth factors (a and bFGF) are closely related peptides that act as potent mitogens and differentiation factors for a wide variety of mesoderm and neuroectoderm derived cells.[1,2] Basic FGF (bFGF pI = 9.6) was first identified by its ability to cause the proliferation and phenotypic transformation of BALB-C 3T3 fibroblasts.[3] Acidic FGF (aFGF pI = 5.6), in turn, was originally identified by its ability to cause the proliferation and delayed differentiation of myoblasts,[4] and to stimulate endothelial cell proliferation.[5,6] Acidic FGF was definitively characterized by Thomas et al.[7] Basic FGF and aFGF are multifunctional; each can either stimulate proliferation or induce or delay differentiation of cells that express FGF receptors.[8-12] Do FGFs use similar or different signaling pathways to mediate cell growth,[13] differentiation, and survival?[14,16] An obvious expectation is that these complex processes are mediated by diverse and divergent pathways.[17] However, biochemical and genetic evidence has indicated that the same molecules, post-translational events, and strategies are frequently used to initiate and carry out very different responses. An easy, but unsatisfying way to explain this paradox is to invoke a combinatorial mechanism whereby the same signals are used in different combinations to evoke specific functions.[18] While the cellular action of bFGF is exerted through its interactions with cell surface receptors, the mechanisms of transfer of mitogenic and/or other specific signals to the nucleus (leading to the "pleïotropic response" required to bring quiescent cells into full proliferation and/or to acquire a differentiated phenotype) are at present unknown. With the exception of the ligand-regulated enhancers — the glucocorticoid, estrogen, thyroid hormones and retinoic acid receptors — no regulatory pathway has yet been entirely traced through an unbroken chain of identified and characterized components, all the way from a defined extracellular signal to a specific nuclear response, in the form of transcription and/or DNA replication. In this context, nuclear targeting of FGF appeared a particularly attractive model system that could bring crucial progress in the knowledge of the mechanism of action of such growth factors.

# II. FATE OF EXOGENOUS bFGF IN THE TWO TARGET CELLS: ADULT BOVINE AORTIC ENDOTHELIAL (ABAE) CELLS AND SWISS 3T3 FIBROBLASTS

## A. NUCLEAR TRANSLOCATION AND FATE OF bFGF DURING THE CELL CYCLE

Quiescent ABAE and Swiss 3T3 cells provide a good experimental system to study the fate of exogenous bFGF that promotes the growth of these two cell types. The addition of bFGF (1 ng/ml of 155, 146, or 131 amino acid isoforms in culture medium; see Figures 1 and 2) to quiescent sparse ABAE or quiescent confluent Swiss 3T3 cells (20 ng/ml of medium culture) induced transition G1 to S phase of the cell cycle after 2 and 8 h, respectively.[21] The acidic form of FGF is also mitogenic for ABAE cells, but higher concentrations are required for similar response.[22] To follow the uptake of exogenous bFGF by these cells, iodinated bFGF (146 a.a. form) was used to stimulate the cell growth.

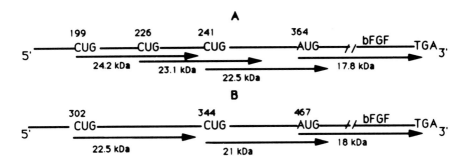

**FIGURE 1.** Partial bFGF mRNA sequence. CUG and AUG indicate the start codons; number above the sequence, its position; arrows, the corresponding forms of bFGF in kDa; 17.8 to 18 kDa = 155 amino acids. (Data from (A) Florkiewicz and Sommer, 1989;[19] (B) Prats et al., 1989.[20])

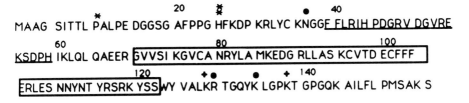

**FIGURE 2.** bFGF sequence of 155 amino acids form.[23] Peptide fragment that stimulates the thymidine incorporation into quiescent 3T3 fibroblasts and modifies basal vascular cell growth in the underlined. This peptide does not bind to the heparin and bFGF receptor.[24] (●) and (+) indicate first and second sulfate ion binding sites, respectively.[25,26] The bFGF sequence important for high biological activity is boxed.[27] * and ** correspond to the 146 and 131 amino acid forms, respectively.

The factor was detected in the cytoplasm (90%) and in the nucleus (10%) of the cells undergoing G1-S transition, as previously observed for exponentially growing cells.[28-30] Basic FGF uptake was continuous in the cytoplasm throughout the cell cycle with a maximum in G2, while nuclear uptake occurred only in late G1. Cytoplasmic bFGF (18.4 kDa) is cleaved into a 16.5 kDa peptide in G1 ($t_{1/2}$ = 30 min). In the nucleus, only the 18.4 kDa form was detected during the 2 h following bFGF addition and then was cleaved into the 16.5 kDa form in the early S phase.[29] These data clearly demonstrate that the intracellular localization of the exogenous growth factor is strictly controlled during the cell cycle and that the nuclear translocation is not related to the cytoplasmic concentration of the bFGF. In order to overcome some of the limitations inherent to a subcellular fractionation procedure, we have also used another independent approach for assaying the compartmentalization of bFGF, i.e., indirect immunofluorescence with an affinity purified polyclonal antibody anti-bFGF.[28] It is noteworthy that, since this approach involves a prior permeabilization of the cell membrane to allow entry of the antibody, an important leakage from cytoplasmic components is likely to take place, making it impossible to evaluate the actual nuclear-cytoplasmic ratio in these conditions. However, this approach confirms the results obtained by the subcellular fractionation

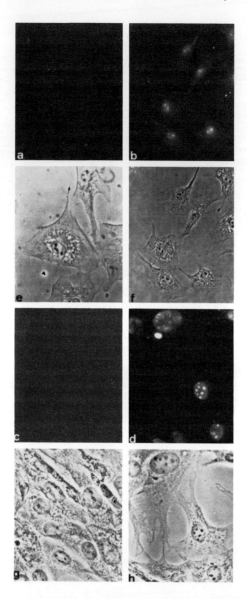

**FIGURE 3.** Indirect immunofluorescence staining of synchronous growing ABAE (a, b, e, f) and 3T3 (c, d, g, h) cells with preimmune rabbit IgG (a); affinity purified anti-bFGF antibody (b, d); and corresponding phase contrast (e, g, h). (Magnification × 220.)

procedure (Figure 3). A bright staining was observed in the nucleoli, with a diffuse staining of the nucleoplasmic network and the cytoplasm of synchronously growing ABAE and 3T3 cells.

The localization of bFGF in the nucleolus was achieved by electron microscopy after immunoreaction using colloidal gold labeled anti-rabbit IgG.[31] It is largely associated with the fibrillar components which correspond to the site of rRNA synthesis.[32] In addition, significant labeling of the nucleoplasmic network was also observed.

## B. NUCLEAR TARGETS OF bFGF

In previous work, we showed that cell cycle dependent uptake of bFGF is correlated both *in vivo* and *in vitro* to an overall stimulation of transcription, and, more specifically, to an increased transcription of genes coding for ribosomal RNA (rDNA).[28] This raised the possibility that bFGF could act on rDNA transcription, either by binding directly to DNA regulatory sequences or as part of a trans-acting multimeric complex. More recently, we showed[30] that bFGF recognizes the 3′ to 5′ lower strand ($GT_{28}$) of a 56 bp putative Z-DNA sequence located upstream the spacer promoter of rRNA genes (Figure 4). This location suggests that the bFGF binding site could act as a regulatory element mediating bFGF enhancement of rDNA transcription by modifying local DNA topology. The transcriptionally induced changes in DNA supercoiling raise the attractive possibility that local variations in superhelicity may exist depending on the position of the promoters, the rate of transcription, and the distribution of topoisomerases. A particular genetic locus in eukaryotic cells could become supercoiled at a particular stage of cellular life. This provide a way for transcription of a given gene to regulate adjacent gene via DNA topology involving a spatio-temporal coordination of transcription patterns of genes.[34] The chromosomic organization of rRNA genes repeated in tandem gives this possibility. Recent findings suggest also that bFGF can regulate transcription directly in the nucleus in a gene-specific manner.[35]

## III. NUCLEAR LOCALIZATION OF ENDOGENOUS bFGF

Some human, rodent, and bovine cell lines[36-40] and tissues[41-44] produce bFGF. In all these cellular species and tissues, endogenous bFGF was detected in the cytoplasm and the nuclei of the cells. Bovine corneal endothelial cells and bovine endothelial cells from the aortic arch and adrenal cortex capillaries also contain detectable bFGF in their nucleoli.[39] Several molecular forms of bFGF are generally synthesized. In the human hepatoma cell line SK-HEP-1, four molecular forms (17.8, 22.5, 23.1, and 24.2 kDa) are co-expressed (Figure 1).[19] The 17.8 kDa bFGF is translationally initiated at the previously predicted AUG codon, whereas the 22.5, 23.1 and 24.2 kDa forms initiate at CUG codons. The higher molecular weight forms are colinear NH2-terminal extensions of the 18 kDa bFGF. Prats et al.[20] have also shown that the *in vitro* transcription-translation of a 6.75 kb human hepatoma-derived bFGF cDNA generated three forms of bFGF with molecular masses of 18, 21, and 22.5 kDa. By use of *in vitro* mutagenesis, it was found that the 22.5 and 21 kDa bFGF forms were initiated with CUG start codons, while the 18 kDa bFGF was initiated with an AUG codon (Figure 1). By transfection into COS cells of intact human hepatoma bFGF cDNA or of a construct from which the AUG initiator was eliminated, it was found that the higher molecular mass forms of bFGF were as biologically active as the 18 kDa form.

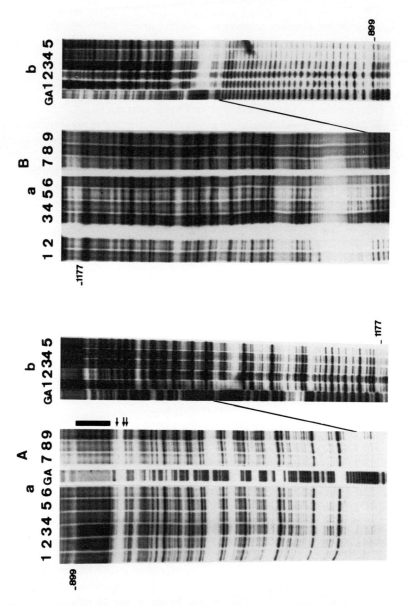

**FIGURE 4.** DNAaseI footprint of bFGF. (**A**) Panel a (lanes 1 to 2): No bFGF; DNA digested with 0.5 and 1 U of DNAaseI, respectively. (Lanes 3, 4, 5, 6): DNA digested with 1 U of DNAaseI in presence of 3, 9, 12, 18 pmol of bFGF, respectively. (Lanes 7, 8, 9): DNA digested with 1.5 U of DNAaseI in the presence of bFGF as in 4, 5, 6. Solid bar alongside the footprint indicates sites protected from DNAaseI digestion in the presence of bFGF. Positions of enhanced DNAaseI cleavage are indicated with arrows. Panel b: Short migration showing the 3' end of the lower strand. (Lanes 1, 2, 3, 4, 5): DNA digested with 1 U of DNAaseI in the presence of 0, 3, 9, 12, 18 pmol bFGF, respectively. (**B**) Panel a: as in A, panel a. Panel b: Short migration showing the 3' end of the upper strand. Lanes 1, 2, 3, 4, 5 as in A, panel b. GA indicates the fragments of the probe produced by purine-specific cleavage. Numbering of the sequence is with respect to spacer promoter of the mouse rRNA gene.[33]

The subcellular distribution of different endogenous forms of bFGF was investigated in cells normally expressing this growth factor[36,37,39,45] and in cells transfected with an expression vector containing the bFGF cDNA.[39,46,48] The subcellular distribution of endogenous bFGF was first studied in the human hepatoma cell line, SK Hep-1.[36] Basic FGF was demonstrated in cytosol, nuclei, and membranes. About 65% of bFGF bioactivity was present in cytosol and 17% in nuclei, while 18% was associated with membranes. Antisera raised against either recombinant 18 kDa bFGF or an N-terminal extension peptide showed that cytosol contained bFGF of mainly 18 kDa, whereas nuclear and membrane fractions contained three forms of bFGF of 18, 22.5, and 24 kDa. Mitogenic activity in nuclei was chromatin-associated and required 0.6 $M$ NaCl or 100 μg/ml heparin for maximal release. The same results were obtained with NIH 3T3 cells transfected with a bFGF cDNA.[45] The cDNA mutagenesis and COS cell expression experiments likewise show that individual isoforms are differentially localized. Nevertheless, data obtained from these various approaches show certain discrepancies. Florkiewicz et al.[46] found that the bFGF forms initiated at CUG codons (i.e., the 22.5, 23.1, and 24.2 kDa isoforms) localize exclusively in the nuclei of transfected COS cells, whether by the four forms together or by one form alone. In contrast, the AUG-initiated 18 kDa form is both nuclear and cytoplasmic. Somewhat different results were obtained by Bugler et al.,[48] who found that, while the CUG-initiated forms are nuclear, the AUG-initiated 18 kDa form is solely cytoplasmic.

# IV. NUCLEAR LOCALIZATION OF ENDOGENOUS FGFs DURING THE *XENOPUS* DEVELOPMENT

Mesodermal induction, the earliest inductive cell-cell interaction in vertebrate embryogenesis, is thought to be mediated by polypeptide growth factors including FGFs.[49-54] In early stages of embryogenesis in *Xenopus laevis,* endogenous FGF[42] is first localized by immunocytochemistry in the cytoplasm of both the animal and vegetal hemispheres of oocytes. After fertilization, however, this localization is altered, and by the eight cells stage the protein is concentrated in the cytoplasm of marginal zone and vegetal pole. This suggests that FGF is redistributed to become preferentially localized in the mesoderm- and endoderm-forming regions of the embryo. In mid-blastula stages, a change in subcellular distribution of bFGFs becomes apparent at the time of mesoderm induction. During stage 8, the staining patterns of bFGF and aFGF become distinct. bFGF is predominantly nuclear and remains in this location during gastrula and neurula stages. In contrast, aFGF was mainly cytoplasmic at stages 9 and 10, although many nuclei showed some level of immunoreactivity.[42] These authors suggest that the FGFs translocated to the nuclei act as transcription factors activating mesodermal gene expression.

# V. NUCLEAR LOCALIZATION OF ENDOGENOUS ACIDIC FGF

aFGF was originally isolated from nervous tissue where it seemed to be almost exclusively located. More recently, several reports have indicated that aFGF was more widely distributed and that large amounts of aFGF could also be localized and purified from other sources, such as kidney or heart.[55] The first nuclear localization of aFGF was described by Sano et al..[56] Then, several works of Courtois' group described the presence of aFGF in the nucleus of corneal epithelium,[57] in the nucleus of photoreceptors of the retina and of astrocytes of the optic nerve of several mammals,[58-60] and in the nucleus of mouse myofibers.[61] Nuclear translocation of aFGF is important for its biological responses. The aFGF NH2-terminal domain contains the sequence NYKKPKL (residues 21 to 27), which is similar to nuclear translocation sequences of other nuclear proteins.[62] Polymerase chain reaction mutagenesis and prokaryotic expression systems were used to prepare a mutant lacking this putative nuclear translocation sequence. This mutant retains its ability to bind to heparin but fails to induce DNA synthesis and cell proliferation. Attachment of the nuclear translocation sequence from yeast histone 2B at the amino terminus of this mutant yields a chimeric polypeptide with mitogenic activity.[63]

# VI. HOW bFGF ACCUMULATES IN THE NUCLEUS OF TARGET CELLS

How bFGF accumulates in the nucleus is unclear. The bFGF isoforms do not contain a short run of consecutive aminoacids which function as nuclear targeting signals in other proteins (SV-40 T-antigen, *Xenopus* nucleoplasmin, yeast histone H2B), while the aFGF contains a putative nuclear localization sequence.[63] Nonetheless, Quarto et al.[47] report that the nuclear localization of the endogenous higher molecular weight forms of bFGF derives specifically from the amino acid sequences within the NH2-terminal extension. However, it is not immediately apparent whether the extended amino terminal domains of CUG-initiated forms functionally constitute bFGF targeting signals, because the endogenous AUG-initiated form which does not include these sequences is also found in the nucleus.[45,46]

bFGF is a signaling protein, as are other known growth factors and peptide hormones. Hence its nuclear targeting probably does not follow the classical scheme[64] described for the import of structural proteins into the nucleus and the nucleolus, and that may account generally for a continuous flow between the cytoplasm and the nucleus. Three lines of evidence argue in favor of a nuclear-specific and discontinuous nuclear uptake of exogenous and endogenous bFGF. Firstly, the translocation of exogenous bFGF[21] and of aFGF[22] is phase-specific during the cell cycle in bovine aortic endothelial cells. Secondly, endogenous bFGF is only detected by immunofluorescence in approximately 10% of the nuclei of interphasic of cultured fetal cardiomyocytes in culture.[37] To explain the presence of the growth factor in a fraction of the nuclei, the authors suggest that the anti-bFGF staining corresponds to cardiomyocytes that are actively synthesizing DNA and are about to undergo mitotic division. Thirdly, FGFs are prepositioned within the *Xenopus* egg in association with yolk in the vegetal hemisphere. They retain this distribution during cleavage and shift subcellular compartments from cytoplasm to nucleus in cells of marginal zone at the time of mesoderm induction during the mid-blastula transition of *Xenopus* development.[42]

Signaling pathways leading to specific transcriptional responses from cell surface ligands must retain the specificity inherent in ligand-receptor interactions. This strict connection between receptor and gene might be carried out through specific protein-protein interactions corresponding to the route taken by FGF between the plasma membrane receptors and the nucleus of the target cells, a route different from the classical pathway through receptor internalization and endocytosis used for cytoplasmic uptake. Several observations favor this hypothesis. bFGF localizes into the nucleus in full length form whereas the cytoplasmic molecules of bFGF are quickly processed.[29,65] The uncoupling of cytoplasmic and nuclear uptakes was achieved by addition of chloroquine to the culture medium of ABAE cells. Nuclear transport was increased by a factor of 2 to 3, while the uptake of the 18.4 kDa form to the cytoplasm was significantly decreased, as was the processing of the 18.4 kDa to the 16.5 kDa form. This result suggests that the cytoplasmic maturation of bFGF occurs in lysosomes. The process of bFGF internalization was also followed in the presence of cycloheximide. The drug was added to the culture medium of quiescent cells together with bFGF. A 50% drop in the cytoplasmic uptake was observed after 2 h, while the nuclear uptake was unaffected.[21] In previous ligand blotting experiments,[66] we showed that the bFGF interacts specifically with 32 to 35 kDa proteins both in the nuclear and the cytoplasmic compartment of growing cells. Conversely, these proteins are not detected in the nucleus of quiescent confluent cells. These results were in agreement with the subcellular localization observed in growing and quiescent cells using exogenous [125]I-bFGF.[29] In the latter case, exogenous bFGF was not translocated to the nucleus.

We propose a model connecting the classical signaling pathway for exogenous bFGF and its cell cycle specific nuclear translocation in growing cells (Figure 5). The exogenous bFGF interacts with several classes of plasma membrane receptors in target cells: high[8-10] and low affinity receptors (heparan-sulfate proteoglycan and/or cysteine-rich bFGF receptors[67]). The interaction of bFGF with high affinity receptor results in an activation of the receptors tyrosine kinase function. The bFGF acting through its receptor tyrosine kinase induces a set of early responses detected within seconds at the level of membranes, or within minutes for cytoplasm and nuclei, resulting in the activation of several cytoplasmic kinases.[17] Concomitantly, the bFGF was internalized via low affinity receptors and interacts specifically with 32 to 35 kDa proteins that probably translocate the growth factor to the nucleus in a cell cycle dependent manner. The 32 to 35 kDa proteins are present in the nucleus and in the cytoplasm of the growing ABAE and 3T3 cells, but only in the cytoplasm of the non dividing cells.[66] Thus the 32 to 35 kDa proteins exist in the quiescent cells in a post-translational state that does not permit its nuclear import and/or is sequestered in the cytoplasm by interactions with another inhibitory protein. The kinases activated by the bFGF-high affinity receptor interaction may modify whether directly or indirectly the 32 to 35 kDa, the inhibitory protein, or both, permitting the 32 to 35 kDa proteins to enter the nucleus. The bFGF interacting with the high affinity receptor was also internalized, but previous experiments[21] suggest that it is degraded in lysosomes.

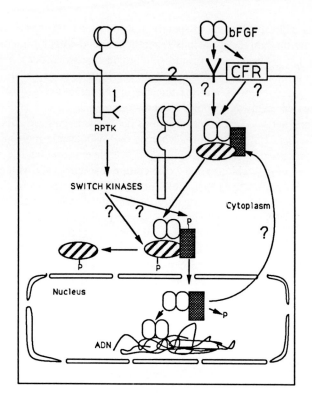

**FIGURE 5.**  The exogenous bFGF nuclear import, a putative model. bFGF interacts as dimer with high-affinity receptors (1), and the resulting activation of receptor tyrosine kinases (RPTK) is transmitted to cytoplasmic kinases.[17] The interacting high-affinity receptors are also internalized (2).[21] Y = low-affinity receptors, CFR = cysteine-rich receptors,[67] ⬭ = inhibitory protein(s), ▓ = 32 to 35 kDa proteins, P = phosphate residues.

# REFERENCES

1. **Gospodarowicz, D., Neufeld, G., and Schweigerer, L.,** Fibroblast growth factor: structural and biological properties, *J. Cell. Physiol.,* 5, 15, 1987.
2. **Burgess, W. H. and Maciag, T.,** The heparin-binding (fibroblast) growth factor family of proteins, *Annu. Rev. Biochem.,* 58, 575, 1989.
3. **Gospodarowicz, D.,** Localization of fibroblast growth factor and its effect alone and with hydrocortisone on 3T3 cell growth, *Nature,* 249, 123, 1974.
4. **Gospodarowicz, D., Weseman, F., and Moran, J.,** Presence in the brain of a mitogenic agent distinct from fibroblast growth factor that promotes the proliferation of myoblasts in low density culture, *Nature,* 256, 216, 1975.
5. **Maciag, R., Cerundolo, J., Isley, S., Kelley, P. R., and Forand, R.,** An endothelial cell growth factor from bovine hypothalamus: identification and partial characterization, *Proc. Natl. Acad. Sci. U.S.A.,* 76, 5674, 1979.

6. **Lemmon, S. K., Rielly, M. C., Thomas, K. A., Hoover, G. A., Maciag, T., and Bradshaw, R.,** Bovine fibroblast growth factor: comparison of brain and pituitary preparations, *J. Cell Biol.,* 95, 162, 1982.

7. **Thomas, G., Rios-Candelore, M., and Fitzpatrick, S.,** Purification and characterization of acidic fibroblast growth factor from bovine brain, *Proc. Natl. Acad. Sci. U.S.A.,* 81, 357, 1984.

8. **Lee, P. L., Johnson, D. E., Cousens, L. S., Fried, V. A., and Williams, L. T.,** Purification and complementary DNA cloning of a receptor for basic fibroblast growth factor, *Science,* 245, 57, 1989.

9. **Reid, H. H., Wilks, A. F., and Bernard, O.,** Two forms of basic fibroblast growth factor receptor-mRNA are expressed in the developing mouse brain, *Proc. Natl. Acad. Sci. U.S.A.,* 87, 1596, 1990.

10. **Dionne, C. A., Crumley, G., Bellot, F., Kaplow, J. M., Searfoss, G., Ruta, M., Burgess, W. H., Jaye, M., and Schlessinger, J.,** Cloning and expression of two distinct high-affinity receptors cross-reacting with acidic and basic fibroblast growth factor, *EMBO J.,* 9, 2685, 1990.

11. **Yayon, A., Klagsbrun, M., Esko, J. D., Leder, P., and Ornitz, D.,** Cell surface heparin-like molecules are required for binding of basic fibroblast growth factor to its high affinity receptor, *Cell,* 64, 841, 1991.

12. **Rapraeger, A. C., Krufka, A., and Olwin, B. B.,** Requirement of heparan sulfate for bFGF-mediated fibroblast growth and myoblast differentiation, *Science,* 252, 1706, 1991.

13. **Gospodarowicz, D.,** Biological activities of fibroblast growth factors, *Ann. N.Y. Acad. Sci.,* 638, 1, 1991.

14. **Schubert, D., Ling, N., and Baird, A.,** Multiple influences of a heparin-binding growth factor on neuronal development, *J. Cell Biol.,* 104, 635, 1987.

15. **Kimelman, D.,** The role of fibroblast growth factor in early *Xenopus* development, *Ann. N.Y. Acad. Sci.,* 638, 275, 1991.

16. **Tamm, I., Kikuchi, T., and Zychlinsky, A.,** Acidic and basic fibroblast growth factors are survival factors with distinctive activity in quiescent BALB/c 3T3 murine fibroblasts, *Proc. Natl. Acad. Sci. U.S.A.,* 88, 3372, 1991.

17. **Paris, S. and Pouysségur, J.,** Mitogenic effects of fibroblast growth factors in cultured fibroblasts, *Ann. N.Y. Acad. Sci.,* 638, 139, 1991.

18. **Chao, M. V.,** Growth factor signaling: where is the specificity?, *Cell,* 68, 995, 1992.

19. **Florkiewicz, R. Z. and Sommer, A.,** Human basic fibroblast growth gene encodes four polypeptides: three initiate translation from non-AUG codons, *Proc. Natl. Acad. Sci. U.S.A.,* 86, 3978, 1989.

20. **Prats, H., Kaghad, M., Prats, A. C., Klagsbrun, M., Lelias, J. M., Liauzun, P., Chalon, P., Tauber, J. P., Amalric, F., Smith, J. A., and Caput, D.,** High molecular forms of basic fibroblast growth factor are initiated by alternative CUG codons, *Proc. Natl. Acad. Sci. U.S.A.,* 86, 1836, 1989.

21. **Amalric, F., Baldin, V., Bosc-Bierne, I., Bugler, B., Couderc, B., Guyader, M., Patry, V., Prats, H., Roman, A. M., and Bouche, G.,** Nuclear translocation of basic fibroblast growth factor, *Ann. N.Y. Acad. Sci.,* 638, 127, 1991.

22. **Bouche, G.,** unpublished data, 1990.

23. **Abraham, J. A., Whang, J. L., Tumolo, A., Mergia, A., Friedman, J., Gospodarowicz, D., and Fiddes, J. C.,** Human basic fibroblast growth factor: nucleotide sequence and genomic organization, *EMBO J.,* 5, 2523, 1986.

24. **Baird, A., Schubert, D., Ling, N. and Guillemin, R.,** Receptor- and heparin-binding domains of basic fibroblast growth factor, *Proc. Natl. Acad. Sci. U.S.A.,* 85, 2324, 1988.

25. **Eriksson, A. E., Cousens, L. S., Weaver, L. H., and Matthews, B. W.,** Three-dimensional structure of human basic fibroblast growth factor, *Proc. Natl. Acad. Sci. U.S.A.,* 88, 3441, 1991.

26. **Zhang, J., Cousens, L. S., Barr, P. J., and Sprang, S. R.,** Three-dimensional structure of human basic fibroblast growth factor, a structural homolog of interleukin 1B, *Proc. Natl. Acad. Sci. U.S.A.,* 88, 3446, 1991.

27. **Seddon, A., Decker, M., Muller, T., Armellino, D., Kovesdi, I., Gluzman, J., and Bohlen, P.**, Structure/activity relationships in basic FGF, *Ann. N.Y. Acad. Sci.*, 638, 98, 1991.

28. **Bouche, G., Gas, N., Prats, H., Baldin, V., Tauber, J. P., Teissié, J., and Amalric, F.**, Basic fibroblast growth factor enters the nucleolus and stimulates the transcription of ribosomal genes in ABAE cells undergoing G0-G1 transition, *Proc. Natl. Acad. Sci. U.S.A.*, 84, 6770, 1987.

29. **Baldin, V., Roman, A. M., Bosc-Bierne, I., Amalric, F., and Bouche, G.**, Translocation of bFGF to the nucleus is G1 phase cell cycle specific in bovine aortic endothelial cells, *EMBO J.*, 9, 1511, 1990.

30. **Roman, A. M., Guyader, M., Truchet, I., Creancier, L., Amalric, F., and Bouche, G.**, Nuclear bFGF binds to intergenic rDNA sequences in growing 3T3 cells: a new signaling pathway?, submitted.

31. **Gabriel, B., Baldin, V., Roman, A. M., Bosc-Bierne, I., Nouillac-Depeyre, J., Prats, H., Teissié, J., Bouche, G., and Amalric, F.**, Localization of peptide growth factor in the nucleus, in *Methods in Enzymology, Peptide Growth Factors*, Part C, Vol. 198, Abelson, J. N., Simon, M. I., Eds., Academic Press, London, 1990, 480.

32. **Sommerville, J.**, Nucleolar structure and ribosome biogenesis, *Trends Biochem. Sci.*, 11, 438, 1986.

33. **Kuhn, A. and Grummt, I.**, A novel promoter in the mouse rDNA spacer is active *in vivo* and *in vitro*, *EMBO J.*, 6, 3487, 1987.

34. **Rahmouni, A. R. and Wells, R. D.**, Direct evidence for the effect of transcription on local DNA supercoiling *in vivo*, *J. Mol. Biol.*, 223, 131, 1992.

35. **Nakanishi, Y., Kihara, K., Mizuno, K., Masamune, Y., Yoshitake, Y., and Nishikawa, Y.**, Direct effect of basic fibroblast growth factor on gene transcription in a cell-free system, *Proc. Natl. Acad. Sci. U.S.A.*, 89, 5216, 1992.

36. **Brigstock, D. R., Sasse, J., and Klagsbrun, M.**, Subcellular distribution of basic fibroblast growth factor in human hepatoma cells, *Growth Factors*, 4, 189, 1991.

37. **Kardami, E., Liu, L., and Doble, B. W.**, Basic fibroblast growth factor in cultured cardiac myocytes, *Ann. N.Y. Acad. Sci.*, 638, 244, 1991.

38. **Hannan, R. L., Kourembanas, S., Flanders, K., Rogelj, S., Roberts, A., Faller, D., and Klagsbrun, M.**, Endothelial cells synthesize basic fibroblast growth factor and transforming growth factor beta, *Growth Factors*, 1, 7, 1988.

39. **Tessler, S. and Neufeld, G.**, Basic fibroblast growth factor accumulates in the nuclei of various bFGF-producing cell types, *J. Cell. Physiol.*, 145, 310, 1990.

40. **Dell'Era, P., Presta, M., and Ragnotti, G.**, Nuclear localization of endogenous basic fibroblast growth factor in cultured endothelial cells, *Exp. Cell Res.*, 192, 505, 1991.

41. **Kardami, E. and Fandrich, R. R.**, Basic fibroblast growth factor in atria and ventricles of the vertebrate heart, *J. Cell Biol.*, 109, 1865, 1989.

42. **Shiurba, R. A., Jing, N., Sakakura, T., and Godsave, S. F.**, Nuclear translocation of fibroblast growth factor during *Xenopus* mesoderm induction, *Development*, 113, 487, 1991.

43. **Woodward, W. R., Nishl, R., Meshul, C. K., Williams, T. E., Coulombe, M., and Eckenstein, F. P.**, Nuclear and cytoplasmic localization of basic fibroblast growth factor in astrocytes and CA2 hippocampal neurons, *J. Neurosci.*, 12, 142, 1992.

44. **Brigstock, D. R., Klagsbrun, M., Sasse, J., Farber, P. A., and Iberg, N.**, Species-specific high molecular weight forms of basic fibroblast growth factor, *Growth Factors*, 4, 45, 1990.

45. **Renko, M., Quarto, N., Morimoto, T., and Rifkin, D. B.**, Nuclear and cytoplasmic localization of different basic fibroblast growth factor species, *J. Cell. Physiol.*, 144, 108, 1990.

46. **Florkiewicz, R. Z., Baird, A., and Gonzalez, A. M.**, Multiple forms of bFGF: differential nuclear and cell surface localization, *Growth Factors*, 4, 265, 1991.

47. **Quarto, N., Finger, F. P., and Rifkin, D. B.**, The $NH_2$-terminal extension of high molecular weight bFGF is a nuclear targeting signal, *J. Cell. Physiol.*, 147, 311, 1991.

48. **Bugler, B., Amalric, F., and Prats, H.**, Alternative initiation of translation determines cytoplasmic or nuclear localization of bFGF, *Mol. Cell. Biol.*, 11, 573, 1991.

49. **Kimelman, D. and Kirschner, M.**, Synergistic induction of mesoderm by FGF and TGF-B and the identification of an mRNA coding for FGF in early *Xenopus* embryo, *Cell*, 51, 869, 1987.

50. **Kimelman, D., Abraham, J. A., Haaparanta, T., Palisi, T. M., and Kirschner, M. W.**, The presence of fibroblast growth factor in the frog egg: its role as a natural mesoderm inducer, *Science*, 242, 1053, 1988.

51. **Kimelman, D. and Kirschner, M.**, An antisense mRNA directs the covalent modification of the transcript encoding fibroblast growth factor in *Xenopus* oocytes, *Cell*, 59, 687, 1989.

52. **Slack, J. M. W., Darlington, B. G., Heath, J. K., and Godsave, S. F.**, Mesoderm induction in early *Xenopus* embryos by heparin-binding growth factors, *Nature*, 326, 197, 1987.

53. **Slack, J. M. W., Isaacs, H. V., and Darlignton, B. G.**, Inductive effects of fibroblast growth factor and lithium ion on blastula ectoderm, *Development*, 103, 581, 1988.

54. **Amaya, E., Musci, T. J., and Kirschner, M. W.**, Expression of a dominant negative mutant of the FGF receptor disrupts mesoderm formation in *Xenopus* embryos, *Cell*, 66, 257, 1991.

55. **Barritault, D., Groux-Muscatelli, B., Caruelle, D., Voisin, M. C., Chopin, D., Palcy, S., and Caruelle, J. P.**, afGF content increases with malignancy in human chondrosarcoma and bladder cancer, *Ann. N.Y. Acad. Sci.*, 638, 387, 1991.

56. **Sano, H., Forough, R., Maier, J. A. M., Case, J. P., Jackson, A., Engleka, K., Maciag, T., and Wilder, R. L.**, Detection of high levels of heparin binding growth factor-1 (acidic fibroblast growth factor) in inflammatory arthritic joints, *J. Cell Biol.*, 110, 1417, 1990.

57. **Dabin, I. and Courtois, Y.**, Acidic fibroblast growth factor overexpression in corneal epithelial wound healing, *Growth Factors*, 5, 129, 1991.

58. **Jacquemin, E., Halley, C., Alterio, J., Laurent, M., Courtois, Y., and Jeanny, J. C.**, Localization of acidic FGF mRNA in mouse and bovine retina by *in situ* hybridization, *Neurosci. Lett.*, 116, 23, 1990.

59. **Faucheux, B., Dupuis, C., Cohen, S. Y., Tourbah, L., Jonet, L., Raulais, D., Vigny, M., Courtois, Y., and Jeanny, J. C.**, Acidic fibroblast (aFGF)-like immunoreactivity in the optic nerve, *Neurosci. Lett.*, 134, 118, 1991.

60. **Faucheux, B., Cohen, S. Y., Delaere, Tourbah, L., Dupuis, C. P., Jeanny, J. C., Raulais, D., Vigny, M., and Hauw, J. J.**, Macroglial cell localization of acidic fibroblast growth factor (aFGF or FGF 1) like immunoreactivity in the optic nerve of young and aged adult mammals, *Gerontology*, 38, 308, 1992.

61. **Oliver, L., Raulais, D., and Vigny, M.**, Expression of acidic fibroblast growth factor (aFGF) in developing normal and dystrophic (mdx) mouse muscles. Distribution in degenerating and regenerating mdx myofibres, *Growth Factors*, 7, 97, 1992.

62. **Dang, C. V. and Lee, W. M. F.**, Nuclear and nucleolar targeting sequences of c-*erb*-A, c-*myb*, N-*myc*, p53, HSP70, and HIV *tat* proteins, *J. Biol. Chem.*, 264, 18019, 1989.

63. **Imamura, T., Engleka, K., Zhan, X., Tokita, Y., Forough, R., Roeder, R., Jackson, A., Maier, J. A. M., Hla, T., and Maciag, T.**, Recovery of mitogenic activity of a growth factor mutant with a nuclear translocation sequence, *Science*, 249, 1567, 1990.

64. **Nigg, E. A., Baeuerle, P. A., and Luhrman, R.**, Nuclear import-export: in search of signals and mechanisms, *Cell*, 66, 15, 1991.

65. **Bikfalvi, A., Dupuy, E., Inyang, A. L., Fayein, N., Leseche, G., Courtois, Y., and Tobelem, G.**, Binding, internalization, and degradation of basic fibroblast growth factor in human microvascular endothelial cells, *Exp. Cell Res.*, 181, 75, 1989.

66. **Truchet, I.**, unpublished data, 1992.

67. **Olwin, B. B., Burrus, L. W., Zuber, M. E., and Lueddecke, B.**, Characterization of a non-tyrosine kinase FGF-binding protein, *Ann. N.Y. Acad. Sci.*, 638, 195, 1991.

Chapter 3

# INTRACRINE ANGIOTENSIN II ACTION

## Richard N. Re

## TABLE OF CONTENTS

0-8493-4713-0/94/$0.00 + $.50
© 1994 by CRC Press, Inc.

# I. INTRODUCTION

The renin-angiotensin system is a well-established regulator of intravascular volume, aldosterone secretion, and arterial vasoconstriction.[1] Renin, an enzyme elaborated by the juxtaglomerular cells of the kidney in response to diminished sodium delivery to the macula densa or diminished perfusion pressure, acts on its substrate angiotensinogen, a hepatically produced alpha-2 globulin, to generate the decapeptide angiotensin I. Angiotensin I is rapidly cleaved by converting enzyme (kininase 2) to the octapeptide angiotensin II. Angiotensin II is a direct vasoconstrictor and a secretogogue for aldosterone. The peptide, in addition, appears to have direct sodium-retaining effects on the renal tubule. Thus, the net effect of activation of the renin-angiotensin system is a tendency towards the restoration of blood pressure and intravascular volume. Much of medicine's ability to interact in a beneficial way with disordered cardiovascular homeostasis depends on its understanding of the physiology of the renin-angiotensin system.

Over the last 15 years, however, it has become clear that in addition to a systemic renin-angiotensin cascade, various components of the renin-angiotensin system exist and, in many cases, are synthesized in tissues.[1-21] This has given rise to the opinion that these local renin-angiotensin systems may subserve physiological functions not immediately apparent from studies of the kidney-based system. In addition, over the last five years an abundance of evidence has accumulated to indicate that angiotensin II can serve as a growth regulatory factor for a wide variety of benign or malignant cell types.[22-43] Thus, it can be hypothesized that regional angiotensin systems may exist either to regulate local blood flow, influence local patterns of cellular growth and differentiation, or, perhaps, serve other functions such as neuromodulation. In sum, then, it now is clear that the renin-angiotensin system, although a fundamental determinant of cardiovascular homeostasis, may well serve additional important roles in specific tissues.

All these studies point up the importance of angiotensin II action in normal and disordered physiology and serve to highlight the question of how angiotensin II acts on its target tissues. It has been clearly established that angiotensin II interacts with specific cell surface receptors now known to exist in the form of at least two subtypes (AT1, AT2) and to influence the metabolism of inositol triphosphate (IP3), diacylglycerol (DAG), and protein kinase C (PKC).[1,2,17,44-46] The mobilization of intracellular calcium stores is a critical step in this activation process and may well serve to link hormone receptor binding with vascular cell contraction on the one hand, and cellular proliferation on the other. In addition, there exists evidence to indicate that angiotensin II binding to its receptor, through the intermediary of G proteins, affects cyclic GMP metabolism, and this signal may be important in the mediation of specific angiotensin II effects.[47] Thus, a considerable amount is known regarding the second messengers generated by this important vasoactive and growth regulatory peptide.

At the same time, it must be recalled that from as early as 1972, data developed by Kharallah and Robertson suggested that angiotensin II could gain access to the cellular interior and translocate to the nucleus.[22] This observation, although for a long time ignored, raised the interesting possibility that the octapeptide angiotensin II could transmit information to the genome in a direct fashion, as do the glucocorticoids and triiodothyronine.

## II. INTRACELLULAR ANGIOTENSIN II ACTION

The original work of Kharallah and Robertson indicated that tritiated angiotensin II, when administered to whole animals, rapidly localized to mitochondria and cell nuclei. Tritiated tyrosine alone did not so localize, and, therefore, these investigators contended that angiotensin II could gain direct access to important intracellular compartments. Unfortunately, competition studies were not carried out, and for a long while thereafter this observation was not pursued. My group, however, decided to confirm and extend the observations of Kharallah and Robertson, realizing that if it existed, a direct intracellular site of action for angiotensin II could have important physiological and therapeutic implications. Originally we isolated nuclei from liver or spleen by standard techniques and confirmed the purity of these preparations by microscopy and standard biochemical assays for membrane contamination. We then carried out standard binding studies utilizing angiotensin II and a variety of peptide analogues for displacement.[48] We observed high affinity specific binding sites, albeit of low abundance, on isolated cellular nuclei. The affinity of binding was approximately 1 n$M$, and the binding affinity of angiotensin II was approximately equal to that of angiotensin III (angiotensin II 2 to 8). Angiotensin I bound 100-fold less well, and it was not clear that some of this binding might not have related to *in vitro* conversion of angiotensin I to angiotensin II. Unrelated small peptides did not specifically bind to the receptors we identified.

In order to follow up on these observations and to further exclude the possibility that undetected plasma membrane contamination could account for our findings, we next employed the tool of DNase I or micrococcal nuclease digestion. A large body of evidence confirms that genetically active chromatin demonstrated enhanced susceptibility to digestion by DNase I or micrococcal nuclease.[49] It appears that nucleosome arrangements are altered in genetically active chromatin so as to provide enhanced access to these enzymes. We treated isolated rat nuclei with angiotensin II and demonstrated that this peptide had the capacity to increase the solubilization of chromatin by approximately $2\frac{1}{2}$-fold.[50-53] This effect was seen at nanomolar and greater concentrations of hormone. Of note, saralasin and the unrelated small peptide, teprotide, were without effect.

In order to further extend these observations, rat liver nuclei (and in additional experiments, thymus-derived nuclei) were digested with micrococcal nuclease following incubation with [125]I-angiotensin II ($10^{-9}$ $M$) in the presence or absence of excess ($10^{-6}$ $M$) unlabeled angiotensin II.[51,52] Chromatin was solubilized using micrococcal nuclease or DNase-1, and after 3 min was applied to a Bio-gel A-5M column. Labeled hormone was 40 to 60% displaceable by unlabeled hormone in nuclear fractions eluting at a characteristic $V/V_0$ consistent with linker DNA. Moreover, a discreet AII binding nuclear protein particle was resolved on DNP gel electrophoresis, and binding to this protein was similarly inhibited by excess unlabeled angiotensin II. Importantly, we observed that micrococcal nuclease digestion in the absence of labeled or unlabeled angiotensin II, followed by exposure of the solubilized fragments to labeled angiotensin II, resulted in no specific binding. That is, specific binding was only seen when micrococcal nuclease digestion occurred in the presence of angiotensin II, suggesting that angiotensin II enhanced the solubilization of its own receptor. This observation is consistent with the hypothesis that the angiotensin II receptor resides in close proximity to genetic elements which are rendered active by direct exposure to angiotensin II. These findings also argue strongly against any possible role of membrane contamination in these results. This is so because any membrane contamination accounting for binding would be present in the preparation, irrespective of whether angiotensin II was present in the incubation mixture.

Taken together, these observations strongly argued for the existence of chromatin-associated angiotensin II high affinity specific receptors which have the capacity of altering chromatin configuration in a way strongly suggestive of genetic regulation. Because of these observations, we concluded that angiotensin II was capable of acting in an intracellular fashion and, therefore, coined the term *intracrine* to mean the intracellular action of a peptide hormone, either after intracellular synthesis or after uptake from cell surface membrane receptors.[52,54] It was, and remains, our view that the intracrine action of angiotensin II and other peptides plays an important role in their physiological function and offers the opportunity for the design of new therapeutic interventions.

In additional studies, we examined the effect of angiotensin II on RNA synthesis by isolated nuclei. At both $5 \times 10^{-7} M$ and $5 \times 10^{-9} M$, angiotensin II significantly increased RNA synthesis by isolated hepatic nuclei.[55,56] This effect was not mimicked by saralasin (Sar[1]-Ala[8]-angiotensin II) or the unrelated nonapeptide teprotide. The exposure of isolated hepatic nuclei to angiotensin II increased RNA synthesis by approximately $2^1/_2$-fold. Of interest, this angiotensin-stimulated RNA synthesis was significantly inhibited by $\alpha$-amanitin, implying that the stimulatory effect was on message-related RNA polymerase II. This finding again suggests a direct effect of angiotensin II binding to chromatin on the transcriptional regulation of specific genes.

Finally, we explored the effects of direct angiotensin II action on the solubilization of divalent cations. We observed that angiotensin II increases the solubilization of copper from chromatin in a dramatic fashion.[57,58] This observation suggests that copper is intimately related to angiotensin II-induced initiation sites and, perhaps, is involved either with the angiotensin II receptor or with the related initiation complex.

In sum, our studies strongly argued for an intracrine role of angiotensin II and raised the possibility that, either after internalization from cell surface receptors of a target cell or possibly after intracellular production by a cell involved in the local or renal renin-angiotensin system, angiotensin II could interact with intracellular sites in a physiologically meaningful way.

# III. CONFIRMATORY OBSERVATIONS

As early as 1988, it had been demonstrated that cells transformed with the *sis* oncogene, which encodes the platelet-derived growth factor B chain, need not secrete PDGF-B into the extracellular medium, but may activate receptors intracellularly, presumably located in the Golgi compartment.[59,60] This, in our view, constitutes an intracrine peptide action, albeit one which is mediated by intracellular second messengers. Of even more relevance to our hypothesis and work, however, was the observation of Rakowicz-Szulczynska et al. that epidermal growth factor (EGF), platelet-derived growth factor (PDGF), and nerve growth factor (NGF) specifically bind to chromatin with high affinity when either intact cells or isolated chromatin are exposed to the growth factors.[61] In addition, this chromatin binding can be blocked by specific monoclonal antibodies directed against the appropriate growth factor receptor, and of even more interest to us was the observation that these growth factors produced a resistance in chromatin to DNAase-2 in the regions in which they bind. These findings are analogous to those we had previously reported for angiotensin II and suggested that all these factors interact with chromatin receptors and thereby regulate gene expression. Yet another common feature between the reports of Rakowicz-Szulczynska and our findings is the fact that the chromatin receptors for NGF, PDGF, and EGF, like our angiotensin II receptor, are extremely tightly bound to chromatin.[61] Also of note is the report that basic fibroblast growth factor (bFGF) enters cells and translocates to nucleoli, whereupon it stimulates RNA polymerase I activity and the transcription of ribosomal genes.[62] These findings again parallel those which we have reported for angiotensin II and its effect on chromatin solubilization and RNA synthesis. Finally, in considering data from other systems, it is noteworthy that intracellular insulin has been demonstrated to stimulate RNA and protein synthesis in *Xenopus* oocytes — results which, again, are strikingly similar to those which we have reported for angiotensin II.[63] Indeed, a similar effect was observed when isolated *Xenopus* nuclei (nuclei which are extremely easy to isolate in a pure state) were exposed to insulin. In this case, once again, a direct insulin effect on RNA synthesis was observed. Taken together, these and other data indicate that the intracrine action of angiotensin II which we have described is likely a common feature of peptide hormone action.[64] This observation is strengthened by still more recent observations. The product of the *tat* gene of the HIV virus functions in a similar intracrine fashion after uptake by target cells as does heparin binding growth factor-1 and interleukin-1.[64-67] These latter two growth factors have been shown to translocate to nucleus and only then to stimulate cell division in target cells. Thus, taken with our original observations, these and other data raise the possibility that a wide variety of peptide growth regulatory factors operate in an intracrine mode.

More recently, our contention that angiotensin II acts in an intracrine fashion has, in large part, been confirmed. Millan and Millan have demonstrated angiotensin localization to the nuclei of target cells.[68] Tang has reported the existence of nuclear receptors for angiotensin II having the same affinity and binding capacity as we previously reported. In addition, this group, using gel shift assays, determined that angiotensin II interacted with the 5′ regulatory region of the renin gene, strongly suggesting a gene regulatory role for this octapeptide.[69] This finding is consistent with the angiotensin II effects on chromatin solubilization and conformation we previously reported. Both results strongly suggest a direct angiotensin II interaction with chromatin resulting in gene regulation. Moreover, Peach and co-workers have reported that in perivascular cells of the kidney — cells capable of generating both renin and angiotensin II intracellularly — angiotensin II can be detected not only in intracellular vesicles, but also in cytoplasm and in nucleus.[70] This result provides powerful evidence that under appropriate circumstances angiotensin II can gain access, through as yet undefined routes, to the nuclear compartment. Finally, Kiron and Soffer reported that an angiotensin II binding species, having characteristics distinct from the cell surface membrane receptor, exists in high abundance in the cytoplasm of a variety of cells.[71] This observation again suggests an intracellular role for angiotensin II and raises interesting parallels between the intracrine action of angiotensin II and the action of steroid hormones.

# IV. CONCLUSION

Abundant evidence exists to indicate that angiotensin II and other peptides can bind to specific high affinity intracellular receptors. Further, data indicates that hormone binding to these receptors appears to be associated in many instances with specific genetic regulatory events. It is plausible, therefore, that these intracrine peptide actions play an important role in normal physiological functioning and possibly in pathophysiological states. Intracrine hormone action provides peptide hormones with yet another means of transmitting specific information to target cells — a mode potentially much less ambiguous than the generation of cascades of second messengers, many of which are shared between a variety of peptide hormones.

The possible function of intracrine angiotensin II action at this time remains speculative. It is tempting to hypothesize that intracellular angiotensin II could play a role in the modulation of cell differentiation and growth which is seen upon exposure of target cells to angiotensin II. Moreover, it may well be that in cells capable of synthesizing components of the renin angiotensin system, a direct feedback of intracellularly generated angiotensin II on the genome may provide a mechanism of regulating the synthesis of the components of the system itself. Given the physiological importance of renin synthesis and secretion in the kidney and possibly other sites, this mechanism should be vigorously explored since it may provide a means of regulating the synthesis of renin and other components of the renin angiotensin system both in the kidney and elsewhere and thereby lead to novel therapies for hypertension and vascular disease.

In sum, considerable evidence exists to indicate that angiotensin II and other peptide hormones can function in what we have termed an intracrine manner. We believe that the intracrine action of peptide hormones is important in determining the physiological actions of these factors and that an understanding of intracrine hormone action will have significant therapeutic ramifications in hypertension, vascular disease, certain neoplasms, and a wide variety of other disorders.

# REFERENCES

1. **Re, R. N.,** The renin-angiotensin systems, *Med. Clin. North Am.,* 71, 5, 1987.
2. **Aguilera, E. P., Hyde, C. L., and Catt, K. J.,** Angiotensin II receptors and prolactin release in pituitary lactotrophs, *Endocrinology,* 111, 1045—1049, 1980.
3. **Ganten, D., Schelling, P., Vecsei, P., et al.,** Iso-renin of extrarenal origin. The tissue angiotensinase system, *Am. J. Med.,* 60, 760—772, 1976.
4. **Felix, D., Harding, J. W., and Imboden, H.,** The hypothalamic-angiotensin system: location and functional considerations, *Clin. Exp. Hypertens.,* A10 (Suppl. 1), 45—62, 1988.
5. **Cassis, L. A., Saye, J., and Peach, M. J.,** Location and regulation of rat angiotensinogen messenger RNA, *Hypertension,* 11, 591—596, 1988.
6. **Re, R. N., Fallon, T. J., Dzau, V. S., Quay, S., and Haber, E.,** Renin synthesis by cultured arterial smooth muscle cells, *Life Sci.,* 30, 99—106, 1982.
7. **Dzau, V. J., and Re, R. N.,** Evidence for the existence of renin in the heart, *Circulation,* 75 (Suppl. I), I134—I136, 1987.
8. **Dzau, V. J.,** Significance of the vascular renin-angiotensin pathway, *Hypertension,* 8, 553—559, 1986.
9. **Eggena, P., Morin, A. M., Barrett, J. D., and Krall, J. F.,** The influence of aging on angiotensin production by rat vascular smooth muscle cells *in vitro, Clin. Exp. Hypertens. Theory Practice,* A10 (Suppl. 4), 597—603, 1988.
10. **Glorioso, N., Atlas, S. A., Laragh, J. H., Jewelewicz, R., and Sealey, J.,** Prorenin in high concentrations in human ovarian follicular fluid, *Science,* 233, 1424—1427, 1987.
11. **Horiba, N. and Nomura, K.,** Effect of exogenous and locally synthesized angiotensin II on adrenal glomerulosa cell growth and aldosterone secretion, program and abstracts of the 70th Annual Meeting of the Endocrine Society, 1988, 102.
12. **Horiba, N., Nomura, K., and Shizume, K.,** Exogenous and locally synthesized angiotensin II and glomerulosa cell functions, *Hypertension,* 15, 190—197, 1990.
13. **Hseuh, Wa,** Renin in the female reproductive system, *Cardiovas. Drugs Ther.,* 2, 473—477, 1987.
14. **Jin, M., Wilhelm, M. J., Lang, R. E., Unger, T., Lindpaintner, K., and Ganten, D.,** Endogenous tissue renin-angiotensin systems from molecular biology to therapy, *Am. J. Med.,* 84 (Suppl. 3A), 28—36, 1988.
15. **Lindpaintner, K., Jin, M., Wilhelm, M. J., Suzuki, F., Linz, W., Schoelkens, B. A., and Ganten D.,** Intracardiac generation of angiotensin and its physiologic role, *Circulation,* 77 (Suppl. I), I-18—I-23, 1988.
16. **Lynch, K., Simnad, V., Ben-Ari, E., Garrison, J.,** Localization of preangiotensinogen messenger RNA sequences in the rat brain, *Hypertension,* 8, 540—543, 1986.
17. **Re, R. N.,** The cellular biology of the renin-angiotensin systems, *Arch. Intern. Med.,* 144, 2037—2041, 1984.
18. **Re, R. N.,** The myocardial intracellular renin-angiotensin system, *Am. J. Cardiol.,* 59, 56A—58A, 1987.
19. **Taylor, G. M., Cook, H. T., Sheffield, E. A., Hanson, C., and Peart, W. S.,** Renin in blood vessels in human pulmonary tumors: an immunohistochemical and biochemical study, *Am. J. Pathol.,* 130, 543—551, 1988.
20. **Buckley, J. P.,** The central effects of the renin-angiotensin system, *Clin. Exp. Hypertens.,* A10, 1—16, 1988.
21. **Suzuki, F., Lindpaintner, K., Keuneke, C., et al.,** Tissue-specific regulation of gene expression for renin and angiotensinogen, *Clin. Exp. Hypertens. Theory Practice,* A10 (6), 1317—1319, 1988.
22. **Khairallah, P. A., Robertson, A. L., and Davila, D.,** Effects of angiotensin II on DNA, RNA and protein synthesis, in *Hypertension,* Genest, J. and Koiw, E., Eds., Springer-Verlag, New York, 1972, 212—220.

23. **Ganten, D., Schelling, P., and Flugel, R. M.,** Effect of angiotensin and an angiotensin antagonist on isorenin and cell growth in 3T3 mouse cells, *Intern. Res. Commun. Med. Sci.,* 3, 327—330, 1975.

24. **Campbell-Boswell, M., and Robertson, A.,** Effects of angiotensin II and vasopressin on human smooth muscle cells *in vitro, Exp. Molec. Pathol.,* 35, 265—276, 1981.

25. **Geisterfer, A., Peach, M. J., and Owens, G. K.,** Angiotensin II induces hypertrophy, not hyperplasia of cultured rat aortic smooth muscle cells, *Circ. Res.,* 62, 749—756, 1988.

26. **Nagano, M., Higaki, J., Mikami, H., Nakamura, M., Higashimori, K., Katahira, K., Tabuchi, Y., Moriguchi, A., Nakamura, F., and Ogihara, T.,** Converting enzyme inhibitors regressed cardiac hypertrophy and reduced tissue angiotensin II in spontaneously hypertensive rats, *J. Hyperten.,* 9, 595—599, 1991.

27. **Naftilin, A. J., Hsaio, L. L., Pratt, R. E., and Dzau, V. J.,** Stimulation of platelet derived growth factor A-chain expression by angiotensin II in cultures smooth muscle cells, *Circulation,* 78 (Suppl. II), II-4, 1988a.

28. **Neyses, L., Vetter, H., Sukhatme, V. P., and Williams, R. S.,** Angiotensin II induces expression of the early growth response gene 1 in isolated adult cardiomyocytes, *Circulation,* 80 (Suppl. I), II-450, 1989.

29. **Baker, K. M., Chernin, M. I., Wixson, S. K., and Aceto, J. F.,** Renin-angiotensin system involvement in pressure-overload cardiac hypertrophy in rats, *Am. J. Physiol.,* 259, H324-H332, 1990.

30. **Pfeffer, J. M., Pfeffer, M. A., Mersky, I., and Braunwald, E.,** Regression of left ventricular hypertrophy and prevention of left ventricular dysfunction by captopril in the spontaneously hypertensive rat, *Proc. Natl. Acad. Sci. U.S.A.,* 79, 3310—3314, 1982.

31. **Campbell, D., and Habener, J.,** Angiotensinogen gene is expressed and differentially regulated in multiple tissues of the rat, *J. Clin. Invest.,* 78, 31—39, 1986.

32. **Linz, W., Scholkens, B. A., and Ganten, D.,** Converting enzyme inhibition specifically prevents the development and induces regression of cardiac hypertrophy in rats, *Clin. Exp. Hypertens.,* 11, 1325—1350, 1989.

33. **Powell, J. S., Clozel, J.-P., Muller, R. K. M., et al.,** Inhibitors of angiotensin-converting enzyme prevent myointimal proliferation after vascular injury, *Science,* 254, 186—188, 1989.

34. **Chobanian, A. V., Haudenschild, C. C., Nickerson, C., and Drago, R.,** Antiatherogenic effect of captopril in the watanabe heritable hyperlipidemic rabbit, *Hypertension,* 15, 327—331, 1990.

35. **Tolins, J. P., Shultz, P., Raji, L.,** Mechanisms of hypertensive glomerular injury, *Am. J. Cardiol.,* 62, 54G—58G, 1988.

36. **Bakris, G. L., Akerstrom, V., and Re, R. N.,** Insulin, angiotensin II antagonism and converting enzyme inhibition: effect on human mesangial cell mitogenicity and endothelin, *Hypertension,* 16 (Abstr.), 326, 1990.

37. **Fernandez, L. A., Twickler, J., and Mead, A.,** Neovascularization produced by angiotensin II, *J. Lab. Clin. Med.,* 105, 141—145, 1985.

38. **Jackson, T. R., Blair, A. C., Marshall, J., Goedert, M., and Hanley, M. R.,** The *mas* oncogene encodes an angiotensin receptor, *Nature,* 335, 437—440, 1988.

39. **Schelling, P., Fischer, H., and Ganten, D.,** Angiotensin and cell growth: a link to cardiovascular hypertrophy?, *J. Hypertens.,* 9, 3—15, 1991.

40. **Chen, L., Re, R. N., Prakash, O., and Mondal, D.,** Converting enzyme inhibition reduces neuroblastoma cell growth rate, *Clin. Res.,* 37, 940A, 1989.

41. **Chen, L., Re, R. N., Prakash, O., and Mondal, D.,** Angiotensin-converting enzyme inhibition reduces neuroblastoma cell growth rate, *Proc. Soc. Exp. Biol. Med.,* 196, 280—283, 1991.

42. **Chen, L. and Re, R. N.,** Angiotensin and the regulation of neuroblastoma cell growth, *Am. J. Hypertens.,* 4 (Abstr.), 82A, 1991.

43. **Chen, L., Prakash, O., and Re, R. N.,** The interaction of insulin and angiotensin II on the growth of human neuroblastoma cells, *Clin. Res.,* 39, 149A, 1991.

44. **Wong, P. C., Price, W. A., Chiu, A. T., Thoolen, M. J. M. C., Duncia, J. V., Johnson, A. L., and Timmermans, P. B. M. W. M.,** Nonpeptide angiotensin II receptor antagonists. IV. EXP 6155 and EXP 6803, *Hypertension,* 13, 489—497, 1989.

45. **Wong, P. C., Price, W. A., Chiu, A. T., et al.**, Nonpeptide angiotensin II receptor antagonists. VIII. Characterization of functional antagonism displayed by DuP 753, an orally active antihypertensive agent, *J. Pharmacol. Exp. Ther.*, 252, 719—725, 1990.

46. **Wong, P. C., Price, W. A., Chiu, A. T., et al.**, Nonpeptide angiotensin II receptor antagonists. IX. Antihypertensive activity in rats of DuP 753, an orally active antihypertensive agent, *J. Pharmacol. Exp. Ther.*, 252, 726—732, 1990.

47. **Langlois, D., Hinsch, K. D., Saez, J. M., and Begeot, M.**, Stimulatory effect of insulin and insulin-like growth factor I on $G_i$ proteins and angiotensin II-induced phosphoinositide breakdown in cultured bovine adrenal cells, *Endocrinology*, 126, 1867—1872, 1990.

48. **Re, R. N., MacPhee, A. A., and Fallon, J. T.**, Specific nuclear binding of angiotensin II, *Clin. Sci.*, 61, 245s—247s, 1981.

49. **Bloom, K. S., and Anderson, J. N.**, Conformation of ovalbumin and globin genes in chromatin during differential gene expression, *J. Biol. Chem.*, 254, 10532—10534, 1979.

50. **Re, R. N., LaBiche, R. A., and Bryan, S. E.**, Nuclear-hormone mediated changes in chromatin solubility, *Biochem. Biophys. Res. Commun.*, 110, 61—68, 1983.

51. **Re, R. N., Vizard, D. L., Brown, T., and Bryan, B.**, Angiotensin receptors in chromatin fragments generated by micrococcal nuclease, *Biochem. Biophys. Res. Commun.*, 119, 220—227, 1984.

52. **Re, R. N. and Bryan, S. E.**, Functional intracellular renin-angiotensin systems may exist in multiple tissues, *Hypertens. Clin. Exp. Theory Practice*, A6 (Suppl. 10 & 11), 1739—1742, 1984.

53. **Re, R. N., Vizard, D. L., Brown, J., LeGros, L., and Bryan, S. E.**, Angiotensin II receptors in chromatin, *J. Hypertens.*, 2 (Suppl. 3), 271—273, 1984.

54. **Re, R. N.**, The cellular biology of angiotensin: paracrine, autocrine, and intracrine actions in cardiovascular tissues, *J. Mol. Cell. Cardiol.*, 21 (Suppl. 5), 63—69, 1989.

55. **Re, R. N.**, Changes in nuclear initiation sites after the treatment of isolated nuclei with angiotensin II, *Clin. Sci.*, 63, 191s—193s, 1982.

56. **Re, R. N. and Parab, M.**, Effect of angiotensin II on RNA synthesis by isolated nuclei, *Life Sci.*, 34, 647—651, 1984.

57. **Re, R. N., Bryan, S. E., LeGros, L., Brown, J., and Byrne, C.**, Copper-rich nucleoprotein generated by micrococcal nuclease, *Biol. Trace Ele. Res.*, 8, 219—229, 1985.

58. **Saucier, M. A., Wang, X., Re, R. N., Brown, J., and Bryan, S. E.**, Effects of ionic strength on endogenous nuclease activity in chelated and nonchelated chromatin, *J. Inorg. Biochem.*, 41, 117—124, 1991.

59. **Doolittle, R. F., et al.**, Simian sarcoma virus *onc* gene, v-*sis*, is derived from the gene (or genes) encoding a platelet-derived growth factor, *Science*, 221, 275, 1983.

60. **Williams, L. T.**, Stimulation of autocrine and paracrine pathways of cell proliferation by platelet-derived growth factor, *Clin. Res.*, 36, 5—10, 1988.

61. **Rakowicz-Szulczynska, E. M., Rodeck, U., Herlyn, M., and Koproswki, H.**, Chromatin-binding of epidermal growth factor, nerve growth factor and platelet-derived growth factor in cells bearing appropriate surface receptors, *Proc. Natl. Acad. Sci., U.S.A.*, 83, 3728—32, 1986.

62. **Bouche, G., Gus, N., Prats, H., et al.**, Basic fibroblast growth factor enters the nucleolus and stimulates the transcription of ribosomal genes in ABAE cells undergoing $G_0$ $G_1$ transition, *Proc. Natl. Acad. Sci., U.S.A.*, 84, 6770—6774, 1987.

63. **Miller, D. S.**, Stimulation of RNA and protein synthesis by intracellular insulin, *Science*, 240, 506—511, 1988.

64. **Burwen, S. J. and Jones, A. L.**, The association of polypeptide hormones and growth factors with the nuclei of target cells, *Trends Biol. Sci.*, 12, 159—162, 1987.

65. **Frankel, A. D. and Pabo, C. O.**, Cellular uptake of the *tat* protein from human immunodeficiency virus, *Cell*, 55, 1189—1193, 1988.

66. **Curtis, B. M., Widmer, M. B., deRoos, P., and Qwarnstrom, E.**, IL-1 and its receptors are translocated to the nucleus, *J. Immunol.*, 144, 1295—1304, 1990.

67. **Imamura, T., Engleka, K., Zhan, X., et al.**, Recovery of mitogenic activity of a growth factor mutant with a nuclear translocation sequence, *Science*, 249, 1567—1570, 1990.

68. **Millan, M. A. and Millan, J. C.**, Nuclear localization of radiolabeled AII in isolated rat adrenal glomerulosa cells, program and abstracts of the 70th Annual Meeting of the Endocrine Society, 1988, 51.

69. **Tang, S.-S., Rogg, H., Schumacher, R., and Dzau, V. J.**, Evidence and characterization of distinct nuclear and plasma membrane angiotensin II binding sites in rat liver, *Hypertension,* (Abstr.) 16, 323, 1990.

70. **Peach, M. J.**, Vascular localization of components of the renin-angiotensin system, presented at the 44th Scientific Sessions of the Council for High Blood Pressure Research, Baltimore, MD, *Hypertension,* (in press).

71. **Kiron, M. A. R. and Soffer R. L.**, Purification and properties of a soluble angiotensin II-binding protein from rabbit liver, *J. Biol. Chem.,* 264, 4138—4142, 1989.

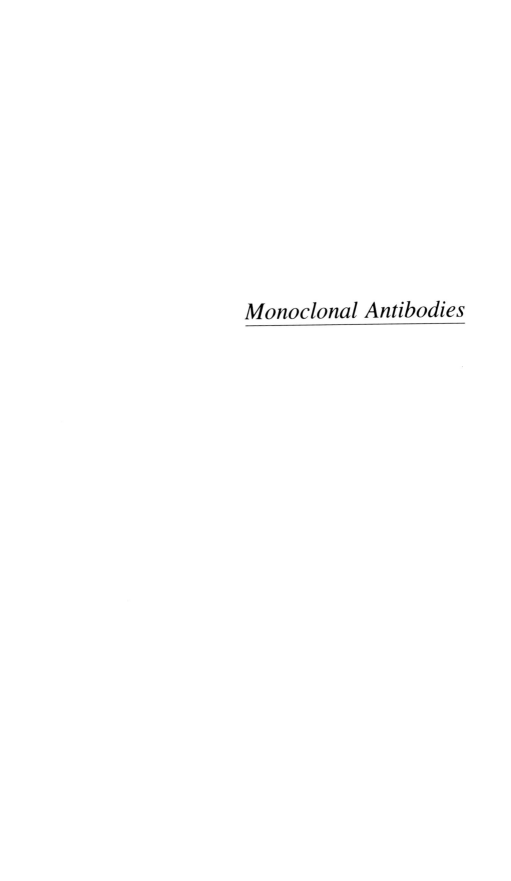

*Monoclonal Antibodies*

Chapter 4

# NUCLEAR ANTIGENS AS THE NEW TARGETS IN CANCER THERAPY

Ewa M. Rakowicz-Szulczynska

## TABLE OF CONTENTS

0-8493-4713-0/94/$0.00 + $.50
© 1994 by CRC Press, Inc.

# I. CLASSICAL APPROACHES TO CANCER IMMUNOTHERAPY WITH MONOCLONAL ANTIBODIES

Monoclonal antibodies (mAb) directed against tumor-associated cell surface antigens have found application in immunodiagnosis and immunotherapy of human tumors.[1-33] Most of the mAb against tumor cells developed in different laboratories recognize blood cell surface antigens (A, B, H, Lewis antigens), HLA antigens, X and Y antigens, related carbohydrates, receptors for growth factors, and differentiation antigens; only a very few are directed against tumor-associated antigens.[34-38] The term tumor-associated antigens is restricted to those glycoproteins and glycolipids that are expressed on the surface of tumor cells and are undetectable or detectable in very small amounts on the normal counterpart of tumor cells or on fetal cells. The existence of antigens of expression restricted to tumor cells is still controversial.[38-40] It is postulated that a sufficiently high density of the antigen on tumor cells compared with a very low expression on normal cells should represent a criticism of diagnostic or therapeutic application of a mAb.[39,40] Most approaches to immunotherapy involve radioactively labeled mAb.[12,13,15,17-21,23] In direct approaches, mAb IgG2a and IgG3 mediate antibody-dependent cellular cytotoxicity (ADCC) in the presence of human effector cells and/or exert complement-dependent cytotoxicity (CDC).[7-9,33,41,42] mAb which inhibit growth of tumors in nude mice provide additional direct cytotoxic effect which can enhance ADCC reaction in the human body.

Mouse mAb injected into cancer patients induce strong immunologic reaction.[43] To diminish the immunological reaction against the mouse immunoglobulin, several laboratories generated human mAb.[44,45] The progress in production of human anti-cancer mAb is slow due to high technical difficulties. Induction of anti-mouse response in patients treated with mouse mAb may also be eliminated by using a mouse-human chimeric antibody.[46-49] Chimeric antibodies are the genetic constructs containing the variable parts of the light and heavy chains of the mouse antibody which determine the idiotypic specificity and the constant region of both light and heavy chains replaced by the human counterparts.[46-49] The immune response of patients to the chimeric mAb is minimal. One type of antibody produced by patients treated with anti-cancer mAb (i.e., the anti-idiotypic antibody) was found to play a beneficial role.[50-52] These anti-idiotypic antibodies that functionally mimic epitopes associated with human cancer cells can induce specific humoral anti-tumor reaction in cancer patients and represent the most specific cancer vaccines.[39]

The parameters which greatly restrict therapy with mAb are low penetration of mAb into the solid tumor, degradation and release from the body, and accumulation of mAb in the liver, kidney, and other normal tissues that express a low level of the same antigen. The basic parameter of tumor cell destruction by the mAb is a sufficiently high density of the target antigen, expressed on the cell surface of tumor cells,[33,42,45] compared to the lowest possible expression of the same antigen on normal cells.

The cell surface density of the target antigen is likely to be much less important when an antibody is internalized into the cell. There are several evidences for the high killing potential of internalized immunotoxins (reviewed in references 53 and 54). Immunotoxins are the mAb with the covalently attached, highly cytotoxic toxins. Conjugates of mAb with two toxins have been tested; diphtheria toxin and ricin, with a predominant use of the plant-derived ricin toxin. Ricin consists of two subunits: A (toxic subunit) and B (cell-binding subunit). In the native form, heterodimeric molecule A-B of the ricin attaches to the cell through the mediation of the B subunit, which involves internalization of the A subunit. For the therapeutic purposes, subunit A, (which, separated from B subunit, is unable to penetrate the cell) is being attached to the mAb which is used as a new vehicle of the A subunit. Internalization of a mAb results in transportation of the subunit A of ricin into the cytoplasm. It was suggested that ricin A inhibits protein synthesis by enzymatically inactivating the EF2-binding portion of the large ribosomal subunit.[55] The recent studies of Endo et al.[56,57] indicated that ricin A inactivates the ribosomes by modifying nucleotide residues ($G_{4323}$ and/or $A_{4324}$) in 28S rRNA. The first immunotoxin was constructed of mAb 17-1A (against colorectal carcinoma-associated antigen) and ricin A in 1980,[58] followed by several constructs containing mAb reacting with tumor antigens[59-65] or various receptors on lymphocytes.[66-72] It was noted that some immunotoxins have poor cytotoxicity.[66,73] Several immunotoxins have been evaluated clinically,[59,65,71] but thus far clearly positive results were obtained with anti-pan T lymphocyte immunotoxins.[74,75] Poor results obtained with immunotoxins are due to poor access to solid tumors, presence of antigen-negative tumor cell mutants, antigen shedding, instability of the conjugate, and rapid decrease from circulation.[76] Improved tumor localization and decreased liver accumulation was observed with the naturally occurring second form of ricin A ($M_r$ 30,000) which contains lower content of mannose than the 33,000 $M_r$ ricin A.[77] Since internalization-ability of mAb used for developing immunotoxins was not tested prior to conjugation with ricin A, it is likely that cytotoxicity of immunotoxin depends primarily on the effectiveness of mAb internalization. Our studies indicate that the internalization-ability of a particular mAb may be precisely tested, before this mAb is used for the direct therapy, radiotherapy, or immunotoxin therapy.[78-81]

## II. NUCLEAR TRANSLOCATION OF INTERNALIZED ANTIBODIES

The hypothetical ideal tumor-killing substance should penetrate the cell, localize to the nucleus, and rapidly destroy the genetic information of the malignant cell. For a long time, the biological dogmas about the intracytoplasmic degradation of internalized antibodies and other protein ligands, like growth factors, eliminated mAb as candidate-carriers for the radioactive or toxic ligands delivered directly into the cell nucleus. The discovery that growth factors penetrate the cell nucleus[82] and bind to nuclear proteins (antigens) recognized by mAb developed against the cell surface antigens[78,83-86] (see Chapter 1) focused our attention on intracellular distribution of internalized mAb. Analyzing the effect of different mAb on tumor cells and following the fate of internalized mAb we made a surprising discovery of nondegraded mAb inside the nucleus of intact cells.[78-80]

## TABLE 1
### Internalization of mAb Directed Against Cell Surface Antigens that Represent Receptors for Growth Factors, Proteins of the Unknown Function, Glycoproteins, or Glycolipids

| mAb | Cell surface antigen | Chromatin antigen | Internalization and nuclear translocation |
|---|---|---|---|
| | *Protein*[a] | | |
| ME 20.4[87] | NGF receptor, 75 kDa,[87] | 230 kDa,[83] 92 kDa,[84] 35 kDa[83,85] | − [86] |
| ME 82.11[87] | NGF receptor, 75 kDa[87] | 230 kDa,[83] 92 kDa,[84] 35 kDa[83,85] | − [86] |
| mAb 425[88] | EGF receptor, 175 kDa[88] | 230–250 kDa[78] | + [86] |
| ME 491[89] | 30–60 kDa glycoprotein[90] | 55 kDa[79] | + [79] |
| ME 49.9[91] | Protein[91] | Detected, not identified[c] | + [c] |
| Anti-breast cancer cells[92] | Protein 80 kDa[93] | 80 kDa[93] | + [93] |
| CO17-1A[94] | 40 kDa protein[95] | Indicated, not identified[c] | + [96,c] |
| GA73.3[97] | 40 kDa protein[95,98] | 37 kDa[c] | + [c] |
| | *Carbohydrate/carbolipid*[b] | | |
| Br 15-6A[99] | Y determinant,[99] 108 kDa,[80] 92–96 kDa,[80] EGF receptor[100] | 88 kDa protein[80] | + [80] |
| Br 55.2[99] | Y, B 108 kDa,[99] EGF receptor[100] | 88 kDa protein[80] | − [80] |
| CO19-9[101] | Sialylated Lewis[a] [101] | Not expressed[80] | − [80] |
| CO51.4[102] | Lewis[a] [102] | Not expressed[c] | − [c] |
| CO29.11[103] | Lewis[a] and Lewis[b] [103] | Not expressed[c] | − [c] |
| CO10[104] | Lewis[b] and H type 1[104] | Not expressed[c] | − [c] |
| CO430[105] | Lewis[b] [105] | Not expressed[c] | − [c] |
| ME 36.1[106] | GD₂/GD₃ Chondroitin sulfate | Not expressed[c] | − [c] |
| ME 313[107] | Proteoglycan[107] | Not expressed[c] | − [c] |
| ME 24[108] | GD₃[108] | Not expressed[c] | − [c] |

[a]   The epitope recognized by mAb is located within a protein domain.
[b]   The epitope recognized by mAb is located with a carbohydrate or carbolipid structure.
[c]   Rakowicz-Szulczynska, E., unpublished data.

We have labeled with $^{125}$I a number of mAb developed against different cell surface antigens expressed on tumor cells (Table 1) and incubated 1 to 24 h with the target cells. A simple pattern was found between mAb internalization and the nature of the cell surface target-antigens; most (but not all) of mAb directed against protein domains of the target antigens were internalized by cells,[78,79] while most of mAb against carbohydrate epitopes were not internalized.[80] mAb against gly-colipids were not internalized. Frequently, a fraction of mAb internalized by the cell was taken up by the cell nucleus and bound to the chromatin. The internalizable mAb immunoprecipitated specific chromatin antigens (Table 1) which are likely to represent nuclear targets for these mAb.[78-80]

## A. MONOCLONAL ANTIBODIES AGAINST CELL SURFACE RECEPTORS FOR GROWTH FACTORS

We have shown in Chapter I that mAb 425 (IgG82a) against the EGF receptor[78] and mAb 20.4 or 82.11 (IgG1), both against the NGF receptor,[87] that were developed against cell surface (plasma membrane) receptors, are able to recognize and immunoprecipitate another antigen-molecule localized in the cell nucleus.[78,79,83-85,102] Since both ligands EGF and NGF, after binding to the cell surface receptors, are internalized by cells and translocated to the cell nucleus,[78,82] in further experiments we tested the steps which follow binding of mAb 425 or mAb ME 20.4 and mAb ME 82.11 to the appropriate receptor localized on the tumor cell surface.

### 1. mAb 425 Against EGF Receptor

Cells were exposed to [125]I-mAb 425 for 1 to 24 h and intracellular distribution of radioactivity was tested. [125]I-mAb 425 was extensively internalized by epidermoid, breast, and colorectal carcinoma cell liens and by normal fibroblasts that express the EGF cell surface receptor (Table 2).[78] Cell fractionation indicated that [125]I-mAb 425 was localized in cytoplasm and in the nucleus (Table 2). It is noteworthy, that mAb 425 was internalized and translocated to the nucleus more efficiently than EGF; for example, in A431 cells, after 1 h of incubation, cytoplasm accumulate twice more and chromatin 5.5 times more [125]I-mAb 425 molecules than [125]I-EGF molecules. Electrophoretic analysis of the [125]I-mAb 425 extracted from the chromatin showed that the mobility of the heavy and light chains of this mAb were the same as those of native mAb (Figure 1). It seems, therefore, that mAb 425 was taken up by the nucleus in a nondegraded form. It is likely that in the nucleus, mAb 425 bound to the 250,000 $M_r$ protein specifically immunoprecipitated by this mAb (see Figure 13 in Chapter 1).[78] The intracellular pathway of mAb 425 is likely to be similar or identical to that of internalized EGF (Figure 2).

### 2. mAb ME 20.4 and mAb ME 82.11 Against NGF Receptor

mAb 20.4 and mAb ME 82.11 against NGF receptor were not internalized by intact cells of the tested melanoma[86] or colon carcinoma cell lines, all of which express NGF receptor and internalize NGF[81,82] (Table 3). Since we found previously[85,109,110] that NGF, after internalization and nuclear translocation, inhibits rRNA synthesis which consequently leads to inhibition of tumor cell growth, we have tested how the cell responds to mAb ME 20.4 or mAb ME 82.11, both of which bind the cell surface receptor but are not internalized and therefore do not interact with the nuclear receptor. In all cell lines in which mAb ME 20.4 or mAb ME 82.11 bound to the cell surface receptor, RNA synthesis measured as [³H]uridine incorporation into TCA-insoluble fraction was 10 to 45% higher than in the same cells not exposed to mAb ME 20.4 (Table 3). In control cell live SW948, which does not express NGF receptors, mAb ME 20.4 did not affect RNA synthesis.

## TABLE 2
### Intracellular Distribution of [125]I-EGF and [125]I-mAb 425 Against EGF Receptor after 1 h Incubation with Intact Cells

| Cell line | Cell or cell fraction | Molecules per cell | | |
|---|---|---|---|---|
| | | [125I]EGF[a] | [125I]mAb 425[a] | [125I]mAb 425[b] |
| *Epidermoid carcinoma* | | | | |
| A 431 | Cell[c] | 850,000 | 790,500 | 670,000 |
| | C | 150,000 | 300,000 | 2,000 |
| | N | 1,300 | 2,000 | 10 |
| | NM | 500 | 1,500 | 5 |
| | Ch | 2,000 | 11,200 | 0 |
| *Breast carcinoma* | | | | |
| SkBr 5 | Cell | 40,000 | 35,400 | 30,000 |
| | C | 10,500 | 8,200 | 500 |
| | N | 250 | 100 | 20 |
| | NM | 700 | 600 | 10 |
| | Ch | 500 | 250 | 0 |
| *Colorectal carcinoma* | | | | |
| SW948 | Cell | 90,800 | 75,000 | 69,000 |
| | C | 65,400 | 62,000 | 1,000 |
| | N | 1000 | 880 | 10 |
| | NM | 200 | 900 | 0 |
| | Ch | 1,250 | 2,950 | 5 |
| SW707 | Cell | 890 | 880 | 785 |
| | C | 330 | 350 | 20 |
| | N | 1 | 2 | 1 |
| | NM | 10 | 5 | 5 |
| | Ch | 35 | 40 | 0 |
| *Fibroblasts* | | | | |
| WI-38 | Cell | 40,500 | 38,000 | 34,000 |
| | C | 26,000 | 29,200 | 850 |
| | N | 220 | 600 | 15 |
| | NM | 120 | 800 | 10 |
| | Ch | 300 | 400 | 5 |

[a]   Incubation at 37°C. Data from seven experiments; SD = 5%.
[b]   Incubation at 0°C. Data from two experiments; SD = 4%.
[c]   Cell = total cell bound; C = membrane-free cytoplasm; N = nucleoplasm; NM = nuclear membranes; Ch = chromatin.

To determine whether ME 20.4 is able to penetrate isolated nuclei, experiments were performed in a cell-free system. [125]I-mAb ME 20.4, when incubated 1 h with nuclei isolated from melanoma or colorectal carcinoma cell lines, was efficiently taken up by the nuclei and bound to the chromatin (Table 3). However, only in those nuclei of HS284, A875 melanoma, and SW707 colorectal carcinoma, all of

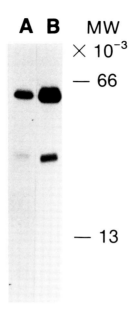

**FIGURE 1.** SDS-PAGE (10% polyacrylamide gel) of [125]I-mAb 425 free (lane 2) and chromatin-bound after 24 h incubation of intact cells. (From Rakowicz-Szulczynska, E., Otwiaski, D., Rodeck, U., and Koprowski, H., *Arch. Biochem. Biophys.*, 268, 456, 1989. With permission.)

which express the specific chromatin receptor (see Chapter 1), was [125]I-mAb ME 20.4 bound to the chromatin (Table 3). Preincubation of isolated nuclei with NGF, followed by incubation with [125]I-mAb ME 20.4, inhibited binding of mAb to the chromatin by 70% (not shown). The obtained results indicate that mAb ME 20.4 is able to penetrate the isolated nuclei and occupies the chromatin receptor for NGF. In nuclei isolated from melanoma WM 164 cells and colorectal carcinoma SW948 cells which do not express the chromatin receptor, mAb ME 20.4 entered the nuclei but remained in the nucleoplasm and did not bind to the chromatin. The latest results prove high specificity of mAb ME 20.4 interaction with the chromatin. To determine the effect of mAb ME 20.4 on RNA synthesis, nuclei were incubated with unlabeled ME 20.4 in the presence of [$^{32}$P]UTP. In the nuclei in which mAb ME 20.4 bound to the chromatin (HS294, A875, and SW707), RNA synthesis was 60% lower, and rRNA synthesis was 55 to 70% lower (Table 3) than in the nuclei not exposed to mAb ME 20.4. In WM164 and SW948, cell nuclei remaining in the nucleoplasm mAb ME 20.4 did not affect RNA synthesis. Thus, activation of the nuclear (chromatin) receptor for NGF by mAb against NGF receptor results in inhibition or rRNA synthesis. mAb ME 20.4 mimics the effect exerted by the original ligand (NGF). However, in intact cells, mAb ME 20.4 is not internalized and therefore selectively activates the cell surface receptor. Both mAb ME 20.4 and

## Internalization of EGF

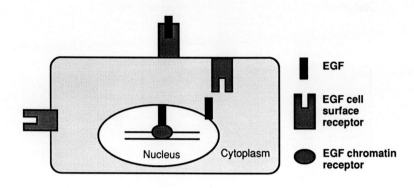

## Internalization of MAb 425

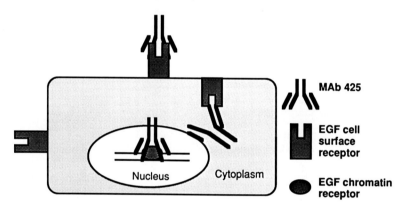

**FIGURE 2.** Hypothetical mechanism of EGF and mAb 425 (against EGF receptor) internalization. Both EGF and mAb 425 are internalized by cell through the cell surface receptor and endocytosis. In the cytoplasm, both ligands are somehow released from the membrane system and penetrate the nucleus. The nuclear, chromatin-bound receptor binds either EGF or mAb 425.

ME 82.11 slightly stimulated cell proliferation. The latest observation confirms our suggestion that stimulation of the cell surface receptor for NGF leads to the second messenger-mediated cell growth activation, while activation of the chromatin receptor results in inhibition of rRNA synthesis, which is leading to the arrest of cell growth (Figure 3).

    Taking into account that mAb to the cell surface antigen may antagonize the inhibitory effect of a growth factor and promote growth of tumors, careful analysis of mAb interaction with both the cell surface and the intracellular antigens should represent a crucial requirement of mAb screening prior to the immunotherapeutic use.

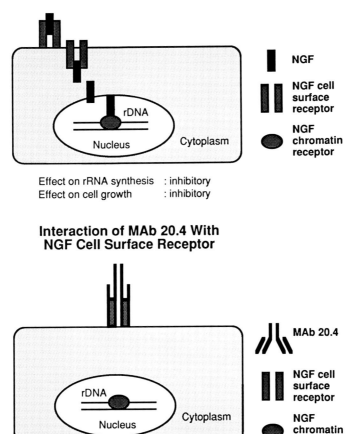

**Interaction of NGF With Melanoma Cell Surface and the Chromatin Receptor**

NGF

NGF cell surface receptor

NGF chromatin receptor

Effect on rRNA synthesis : inhibitory
Effect on cell growth : inhibitory

**Interaction of MAb 20.4 With NGF Cell Surface Receptor**

MAb 20.4

NGF cell surface receptor

NGF chromatin receptor

Effect on RNA synthesis : slightly stimulatory
Effect on cell growth : stimulatory

**FIGURE 3.** Hypothetical mechanism of cell interaction with NGF and mAb ME 20.4 (against NGF receptor). Both NGF and mAb ME 20.4 bind to the cell surface receptor, but only NGF is internalized and translocated to the nucleus. NGF binds to the chromatin receptor which results in inhibition of rRNA synthesis and leads to arrest of cell growth. In contrast, mAb ME 20.4 activates only the cell surface receptor, which promotes tumor cell proliferation.

## B. mAb AGAINST PROTEIN ANTIGENS OTHER THAN GROWTH FACTOR RECEPTORS

Several mAb directed against protein domains of the cell surface antigens different from the known receptors for growth factors are also internalized and translocated to the cell nucleus (Table 1). More advanced studies were concentrated on mAb against a breast carcinoma-associated antigen and mAb[79] against an antigen described as associated with melanoma cell progression.[89,90]

**TABLE 3**

**Uptake of mAb ME 20.4 Against NGF Receptor by Intact Cells
or Penetration of Isolated Nuclei and
Effect on Transcription after 1 h Incubation**

| Cell line | Total cell bound | Cell fraction[b] | | Isolated nuclei | | Intact cells ± NGF | | Isolated nuclei ± NGF | |
|---|---|---|---|---|---|---|---|---|---|
| Melanoma | | | | | | | | | |
| HS 294 | 500,000 | C | 200 | | − | − | 100 | − | 100;100 |
| (NGF·R$_S$, NGF·R$_N$)[d] | | N | 20 | N | 400 | + | 145 | + | 40;30 |
| | | NM | 15 | NM | 580 | | | | |
| | | Ch | 20 | Ch | 10,000 | | | | |
| A 875 | 360,000 | C | 200 | | − | − | 100 | − | 100;100 |
| (NGF·R$_S$, NGF·R$_N$) | | N | 10 | N | 250 | + | 130 | + | 50;39 |
| | | NM | 10 | NM | 700 | | | | |
| | | Ch | 8 | Ch | 5,500 | | | | |
| WM164 | 1,800 | C | 1,000 | | − | − | 100 | − | 100;100 |
| (NGF·R$_S$) | | N | 700 | N | 2,000 | + | 110 | + | 100;100 |
| | | NM | 50 | NM | 600 | | | | |
| | | Ch | 0 | Ch | 100 | | | | |
| Colorectal carcinoma | | | | | | | | | |
| (NGF·R$_S$, NGF·R$_N$) | 3,500 | C | 150 | | − | − | 100 | − | 100;100 |
| | | N | 10 | N | 100 | + | 120 | + | 55;45 |
| | | NM | 2 | NM | 350 | | | | |
| | | Ch | 5 | Ch | 1,000 | | | | |
| SW948 | 100 | C | 50 | | − | − | 100 | − | 100;100 |
| | | N | 0 | N | 1,600 | + | 100 | + | 100;100 |
| | | NM | 0 | NM | 200 | | | | |
| | | Ch | 0 | Ch | 0 | | | | |

Column group header: $^{125}$I-mAb ME 20.4 molecules per cell or nucleus[a] ; RNA; rRNA (%)[c]

[a]   Mean from five to seven experiments; SD < 10%.

[b]   C = membrane-free cytoplasm; N = nucleoplasm; NM = nuclear membranes; Ch = chromatin; mAb ME 82.11 binding to the cell and intracellular or nuclear distribution are very similar to those of mAb ME 20.4.

[c]   RNA — total RNA synthesis measured as [$^3$H]uridine incorporation into TCA-insoluble fraction (intact cells) or [$^{32}$P]UTP incorporation (in isolated nuclei); rRNA — ribosomal RNA synthesis was measured by hybridization of [$^{32}$P]UTP-RNA to the probe of rDNA.

[d]   NGF·R$_S$ — cell surface receptor for NGF; NGF·R$_N$ — nuclear receptor for NGF.

## 1. Quickly and Effectively Internalizing mAb Against a Breast Carcinoma Cell Antigen

*Cell fractionation studies* — $^{125}$I-mAb (IgG2a) was internalized by several breast carcinoma cell lines but not colorectal carcinoma or melanoma cell lines (Table 4). This is the most efficiently internalized antibody we had found until now. On average, 475,815 molecules of $^{125}$I-mAb per cell were cell-associated after 48 h of incubation with MCF-7 breast mammary carcinoma cell line; almost 30%

## TABLE 4
## Internalization and Nuclear Translocation of $^{125}I$ mAb Anti-Breast Cancer Cells after Incubation with Different Tumor Cell Lines

| | | | $^{125}I$-mAb molecules per[a] cell fraction | | | |
|---|---|---|---|---|---|---|
| Cell line | Time of incubation | Cell | Cytoplasm[b] | Nucleoplasm | Nuclear membranes | Chromatin |
| *Mammary carcinoma* | | | | | | |
| MCF-7 | 2 h | 58,337 | 41,710 | 1,500 | 7,627 | 7,500 |
| | 24 h | 220,415 | 171,940 | 6,060 | 16,895 | 25,520 |
| | 48 h | 475,815 | 324,751 | 5,563 | 25,000 | 120,500 |
| SKBr 5 | 2 h | 92,500 | 46,350 | 4,500 | 7,700 | 33,950 |
| | 2 h[c] | 46,950 | 25,200 | 2,000 | 9,400 | 10,350 |
| | 2 h[d] | 16,610 | 6,520 | 590 | 500 | 9,000 |
| | 24 h | 125,010 | 76,140 | 4,260 | 8,790 | 35,820 |
| | 48 h | 115,785 | 69,105 | 1,750 | 7,480 | 37,450 |
| BT20 | 2 h | 4,560 | 2,990 | 100 | 230 | 1,330 |
| | 24 h | 8,770 | 6,180 | 460 | 490 | 1,640 |
| | 48 h | 8,820 | 4,640 | 1,490 | 510 | 2,180 |
| *Colorectal carcinoma* | | | | | | |
| SW707 | 2 h | 6,975 | 2,595 | 200 | 700 | 3,480 |
| | 24 h | 14,290 | 6,760 | 310 | 1,710 | 5,510 |
| *Melanoma* | | | | | | |
| 451Lu | 24 h | 6,720 | 6,420 | 150 | 50 | 100 |
| *T Lymphocytes* | | | | | | |
| SUPT1 | 24 h | 204 | 130 | 42 | 7 | 25 |

[a]  Data from one set of experiments; SD from three experiments is below 15%.
[b]  Crude, membrane-containing.
[c,d]  Cells were first preincubated with unlabeled mAb (100 ng/ml) for 1 h ([c]) or for 24 h ([d]).

were found inside the nucleus, tightly bound to the chromatin (120,500 molecules per cell/chromatin) (Table 4). At the same time of incubation (48 h), another breast carcinoma SKBr 5, accumulated only 115,785 molecules per cell, 37,450 of which were bound to the chromatin. Mammary carcinoma BT20 internalized no more than 8,820 molecules, 2,180 to the chromatin. Internalization and nuclear uptake was also observed in SW707 colorectal carcinoma cells, while melanoma 451Lu bound a low number of molecules to the cell surface only. T lymphocytes (SUPT1) used as a negative control, absorbed mAb on the background level (204 molecules per cell) (Table 4).

It is noteworthy that the kinetics of intracellular uptake and redistribution of mAb were completely different in MCF-7 and SKBr 5 mammary carcinoma cell lines (Table 4). In MCF-7 cells, uptake of mAb increased with time of incubation, being after 48 h 8-fold higher in total and 18-fold higher in the chromatin than after

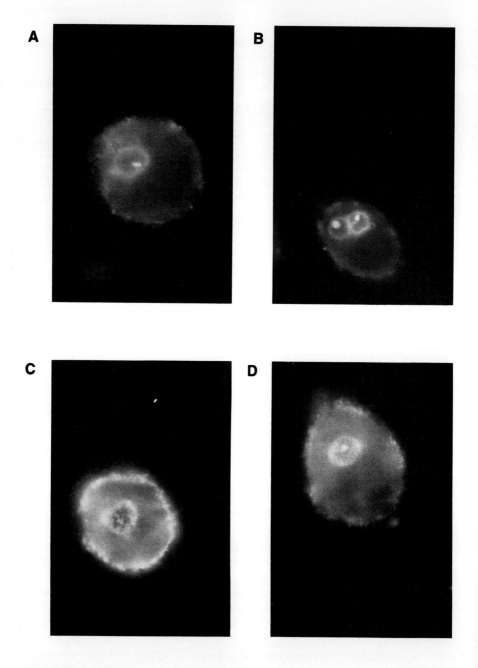

**FIGURE 4.**    Immunofluorescence staining of SKBr breast carcinoma cells incubated 24 h with 20 ng/ml (A,B), 100 ng/ml (C), 500 ng/ml (D) of mAb anti-breast cancer cells with fluorescein-conjugated goat anti-mouse IgG.

2 h of incubation. In SKBr 5 cells uptake of mAb was only slightly higher after 48 h than after 2 h. The different kinetics of mAb uptake and intracellular distribution suggest that the internalization and nuclear translocation are very specific for each cell type and likely to be controlled at the intracellular level.

*Indirect immunofluorescence studies* — Nuclear translocation of mAb in infected cells was also observed by indirect fluorescence staining (Figure 4). After 15 min of breast carcinoma cell incubation with mAb at 0°C, followed by incubation with fluoresceine-conjugated sheep anti-mouse IgG, fluorescent spots were localized in the cytoplasm, which suggest that mAb was internalized and localized in the cytoplasmic membrane system (endosomal pits). After 24 h of incubation with mAb, very sharp fluorescence staining was almost restricted to the nucleolus. A strongly labeled fluorescent ring surrounded the nucleolus (or nucleoli) and a fluorescent spot marked the center of the nucleolus. The distribution of fluorescence suggests that in addition to the membrane-bound antigen, the nucleolus must express the target antigen for mAb.

*Nuclear translocation of mAb in a cell-free system* — Nuclei isolated from MCF-7 breast carcinoma cells were incubated 1 h at 20°C with $^{125}$I-mAb (Figure 5). The amount of the $^{125}$I-mAb translocated to the nucleus was progressively increasing with the increased concentration of $^{125}$I-mAb. Nuclear uptake of mAb was not affected by wheat germ agglutinin (WGA)[111,112] which suggests that the lectin-dependent channel is not involved in recognition of the mAb translocated to the nucleus.

Although the proposed mechanism of mAb "travel" inside the cell is highly speculative, the last step, i.e., chromatin binding of mAb followed by dissociation of the chromatin antigen, seems to correspond to the mechanism of NGF binding to the chromatin receptor (see Figure 38 in Chapter 1). Experimental data suggest that binding of NGF to its 230,000 $M_r$ chromatin receptor results in dissociation of the high molecular weight receptor, leaving a 78,000 to 90,000 subunit bound to NGF. We documented that expression of the low molecular weight subunit of the NGF chromatin receptor is sufficient for NGF binding to the chromatin; however, the inhibitory effect of NGF on rRNA synthesis occurs only after binding to the high molecular weight receptor.[84,86]

*Detection of the target antigens* — Western blotting of proteins extracted from plasma membrane fractions, nuclear membranes, and the chromatin with mAb against breast cancer cells revealed a major, diffuse band ($M_r$ 80,000) and a minor band ($M_r$ 200,000) in all three cellular fractions of MCF-7 and SKBr 5 breast carcinoma cell lines (Figure 6). The 200,000-$M_r$ band was the only one that was detected by mAb in SW707 cells. When the electrophoresis was performed in nonreducing conditions (in the absence of 2-mercaptoethanol), the ratio between the high and low molecular weight protein bands significantly increased (not shown), which suggests that the p80 antigen exists in the form of a monomer and a dimer. In SW707 cells, only the high molecular weight protein was detected in both nonreducing and reducing conditions, which suggests that other than S-S interactions stabilize the high molecular weight form. After a 48-h exposure of the autoradi-

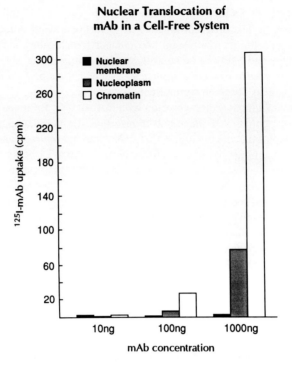

**FIGURE 5.** Nuclear uptake and binding to the chromatin of mAb anti-breast cancer cells after 1 h incubation (20°C). Nuclei were isolated from SKBr cells and resuspended in 0.25 $M$ sucrose, 20 m$M$ Tris-HCl, pH 7.8, 10 m$M$ MgCl$_2$, and 500 ng/ml BSA.

ogram, weak bands ($M_r$ 80,000 and 200,000) were developed in BT20 cells, but not in 451Lu cells.

mAb against breast cancer cells had been until now the only known internalizable antibody able to recognize an antigen expressed in three cellular compartments: plasma membranes (cell surface), nuclear membrane, and in the chromatin. In this respect, mAb against breast cancer cells is unique, since all other internalizable mAb tested recognize electrophoretically distinguishable molecules on the cell surface and in the chromatin and do not recognize any antigen on the nuclear membrane (Figure 5, Chapter 1). The presence of mAb recognized antigens on the nuclear membrane may explain rapid and effective translocation of mAb to the cell nucleus of intact cells (Table 4) as well as the assay excess into the isolated nuclei (Figure 5).

Since the 80,000 $M_r$ antigen was detected in the nuclear membrane, and in the chromatin of cells not previously exposed to mAb, nuclear translocation of the surface antigen in a complex with internalized mAb is unlikely. Adsorption of the cell-surface antigen to intracellular fractions during cell fractionation may be completely eliminated, since other marker antigens of breast carcinoma plasma mem-

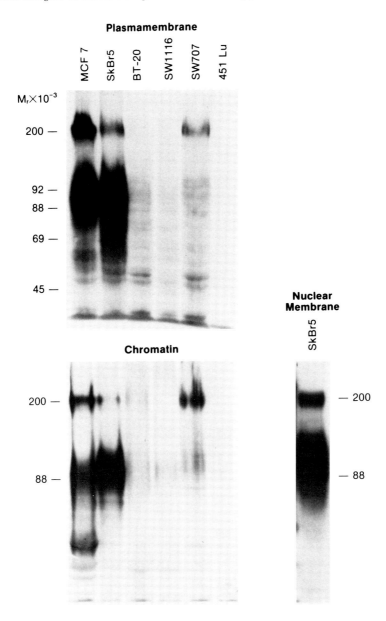

**FIGURE 6.** Western blotting of mAb anti-breast cancer cells with plasma membrane, chromatin, or nuclear membrane proteins of breast (MCF-7, SKBr 5, BT-20), colorectal (SW1116, SW707) and melanoma (451Lu) cell lines separated in a 7.5% polyacrylamide gel and transferred onto the nitrocellulose membrane. $^{125}I$-(Fab)$_2$ fragment of goat anti-mouse antibody was used as the second antibody.

branes such as HIV-1 gp120-crossreactive antigen p160 (see Chapter 2) were not detected in the nuclear membrane fraction nor in the chromatin. It is likely that internalization of mAb into the cell, and then translocation from the cytoplasm to the nucleus, occurs through a cascade system, in which the mAb is first internalized through the cell surface antigen-mediated endocytosis and next released from the membrane system to the cytosol, from which it binds to the nuclear membrane antigen which mediates translocation of mAb across the nuclear envelope. Inside the nucleus, the mAb may be released again and binds to the nuclear antigen. Alternatively, another simple mechanism of mAb "travel" from the cell surface to the chromatin may be anticipated: mAb may bind to the dimeric antigen of the $M_r$ 200,000, which would result in dissociation of the $M_r$ 80,000 protein-mAb complex. If affinity of the 200,000 $M_r$ antigen to mAb is higher than that of the 80,000 $M_r$ protein, then the nuclear membrane-associated antigen may bind the mAb from the $M_r$ 80,000 vehicle subunit of the antigen. The new complex, formed by the nuclear membrane antigen of the $M_r$ 200,000, the mAb molecule, and the dissociated $M_r$ 80,000-mAb complex, is again destroyed inside the nucleus by the 200,000-$M_r$ chromatin (nucleolar) antigen which binds mAb. Dissociation of mAb from the vehicle molecule 80,000 $M_r$ may be dependent on the local variations of pH typical for the particular cell compartments.

*Effect of mAb on RNA and DNA synthesis* — Although the immunofluorescence staining indicated precisely nucleolar localization of internalized mAb (Figure 4), and cell fractionation studies (Table 4) indicated high accumulation of mAb in the nucleus, rRNA synthesis in cells exposed to mAb (1 to 4,000 ng/ml) did not indicate any changes compared to cells not exposed to mAb. Moreover, total RNA synthesis measured as [³H]uridine incorporation into RNA also did not change after cell exposure to mAb (not shown). Nuclear accumulation of mAb in a cell-free system also did not affect RNA/rRNA synthesis. The results clearly show that proteins of the $M_r$ 80,000 and/or $M_r$ 200,000, which seem to represent the nuclear (nucleolar) targets for mAb, are not involved in regulation of RNA (rRNA) synthesis. We cannot eliminate the possibility that some unique genes are affected by chromatin-bound mAb.

mAb, which was used in an unlabeled form (5 µg/ml), did not inhibit SKBr 5 nor MCF-7 cell growth by more than 10%. However, when added to the medium in a radioactive form (¹²⁵I-mAb; spec. act. 20 cpm/pg; 100 ng/ml), it was extremely cytotoxic and killed the cells in 24 h. Chromatin isolated from cells exposed to the radioactive ¹²⁵I-mAb lost the usual viscosity and only partially sedimented during centrifugation by 1.7 $M$ sucrose. DNA, when isolated from cells exposed to [¹²⁵I] mAb showed almost complete fragmentation, as established by electrophoretic analysis and staining with ethidium bromide. The experiments document that the radioactivity emitted by mAb significantly damaged the DNA.

Chromosomal damage after colorectal carcinoma cell exposure to the internalized ¹²⁵I-labeled mAb 17-1A was also described by Woo et al.[96] Since internalization and nuclear accumulation of mAb directed against breast cancer exceeds by 30- to 100-fold that of mAb 17-1A or of other mAb, it is likely that by using mAb, or another mAb internalized in similar quantities, we should be able to decrease the dose of the therapeutic antibody and thereby decrease patients' exposure to the labeled mAb to the minimal level. A mAb that is so rapidly internalized and translocated to the nucleus of tumor cells should accumulate in the tumor and be more harmless to the organism than a slowly internalizable mAb or one which acts only on the cell surface level. Cytoplasmic accumulation of mAb exceeded by threefold nuclear accumulation which also makes this mAb a good candidate for conjugation with ricin A. Effective internalization represents the first criterion of immunotoxic action. Since, theoretically, one molecule of ricin A is sufficient to destroy the cell, the effectively internalized mAb would be potentially best in extremely low concentrations, which should eliminate the toxic effects of ricin A to the minimum.

## 2. Internalized and Biologically Active mAb Against Melanoma-Associated Glycoprotein

In contrast to mAb directed against breast cancer cells (which is accumulated in large quantities in the nucleolus but in unlabeled form does not exert any effect on rRNA synthesis) another mAb — mAb ME 491 (IgM) — directed against a cell surface glycoprotein[89,90] is translocated to the nucleus in much lower amounts[79] (Table 5) than mAb directed against breast cancer cells (Table 4) and without predominantly nucleolar localization (Figure 7), but it does affect rRNA synthesis[79] (Table 6).

*Intracellular localization of* [125]*I-mAb ME 491 by cell fractionation* — Melanoma and colorectal carcinoma cell lines were exposed to [125]I-mAb ME 491 (100 ng/ml) for 1 to 24 h. [125]I-mAb was internalized and accumulated inside the cytoplasm and the nucleus (Table 5). The number of [125]I-mAb ME 491 molecules bound to the chromatin after 1 h of incubation varied from 320 molecules per cell/chromatin in SW1116 colorectal carcinoma cells (lowest internalization), up to 8550 molecules per cell/chromatin in SW948 cells (highest internalization) which corresponds to 8.5 to 22.6% of the internalized molecules (Table 5). Accumulation of [125]I-mAb ME 491 was 25 to 50% higher after 24 h than after 1 h of incubation.

*Intracellular localization of mAb ME 491 by indirect fluorescence staining* — Indirect immunofluorescence staining of SW948 cells with mAb ME 491 indicated mainly cytoplasmic localization with very weak nuclear staining (Figure 7). Inside the cytoplasm, mAb ME 491 was localized in the plasma membranes (endosomal vesicles).

*Specificity of mAb ME 491 interaction with target cell chromatin* — To test whether mAb ME 491 penetrates the nucleus in a nondegraded form, or instead, degraded fragments of [125]I-mAb ME 491 nonspecifically attach to the chromatin, three groups of experiments were performed. In experiment 1, cells were exposed for 24 h to [125]I-ME 491, and chromatin was purified, separated electrophoretically, and analyzed by autoradiography for the presence of [125]I-mAb (Figure 8). Extracted from the chromatin, both heavy and light chains of [125]I-mAb ME 491 showed the same electrophoretic mobility as free [125]I-mAb. The results eliminated degradation of [125]I-mAb ME 491 prior to the chromatin binding.

## TABLE 5
### Intracellular Distribution of Internalized $^{125}$I-ME 491
### after 1 h and 24 h Incubation of Intact Cells

| Cell line | Molecules per cell[a] | | | | | | | | | |
|---|---|---|---|---|---|---|---|---|---|---|
| | Cytoplasm | | Nucleoplasm | | Nuclear membranes | | Chromatin | | % in chromatin | |
| | 1 h | 24 h | 1 h | 24 h | 1 h | 24 h | 1 h | 24 h | 1 h | 24 h |
| SW948 | 27,800 | 32,900 | 800 | 1,000 | 600 | 750 | 8,550 | 8,990 | 22.6 | 20.6 |
| SW1116 | 40,250 | 3,000 | 100 | 200 | 50 | 65 | 320 | 480 | 15.6 | 12.0 |
| WM9 | 26,500 | 35,700 | 400 | 530 | 10 | 10 | 2,500 | 3,800 | 8.5 | 10.3 |
| WM35 | 9,000 | 14,000 | 520 | 600 | 480 | 700 | 1,200 | 2,000 | 10.6 | 11.6 |
| WM983A | 1,580 | 52,000 | 780 | 1,000 | 100 | 150 | 4,000 | 5,800 | 8.9 | 9.8 |

[a]    The mean from three of four experiments (SD = 5 to 10%).

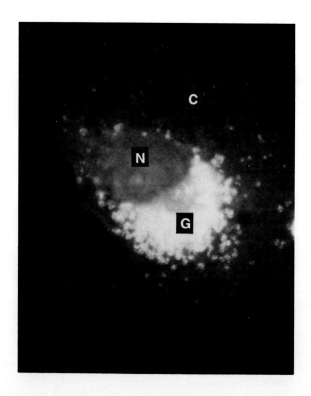

**FIGURE 7.**   Immunofluorescence staining of SW948 cells incubated 24 h in the presence of mAb ME 491 (100 ng/ml) with fluoresceine-conjugated goat anti-mouse IgG. N — nucleus, C — cytoplasm, G — Golgi-associated fluorescence.

## TABLE 6
## Effect of WGA on Nuclear Uptake of [125]I-mAb ME 491 in a Cell-Free System

| Cell line from which nuclei originate | Chromatin-bound molecules per nucleus[a] WGA | | | | |
|---|---|---|---|---|---|
| | 0 | 0.1 mg/ml | 0.5 mg/ml | 1 mg/ml | 10 mg/ml |
| WM9 | 11,000 | 25,000 | 29,500 | 35,000 | 40,000 |
| SW948 | 13,800 | 26,500 | 30,000 | 36,200 | 45,500 |

[a]  Nuclei were incubated 1 h at 20°C in the chemically defined medium containing 0.25 $M$ sucrose, 20 m$M$ Tris-HCl, pH 7.8, 10 m$M$ MgCl, 500 ng/ml (BSA), 100 ng/ml [125]I-mAb ME 491, and increasing concentration of wheat germ agglutinin (WGA). Data are given as means from two experiments; SD = 5%.

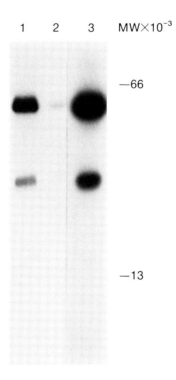

**FIGURE 8.**  SDS-PAGE (10% polyacrylamide gel) of chromatin-bound [125]I-mAb ME 491 after 24 h incubation of intact cells: 12 h exposure (lane 2), 48 h exposure (lane 1), free [125]I-mAb 491 (control) (lane 3). (From Rakowicz-Szulczynska, E. and Koprowski, H., *Arch. Biochem. Biophys.*, 271, 366, 1989. With permission.)

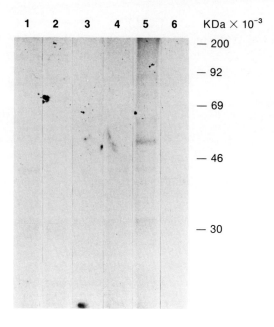

**FIGURE 9.** SDS-PAGE (10% polyacrylamide gel) of chromatin fraction immunoprecipitated from *Hinc*II-digested chromatin of SW948 cells with mAb ME 491 (lane 5), mAb 20.4 (lane 1), mAb 82.11 (lane 2), and control antibody P3 × 63Ag8 (lane 4). In lane 6, chromatin was immunoprecipitated again with mAb ME 491, after the immunoprecipitate (lane 5) was removed by centrifugation.

In experiment 2, we attempted to determine whether [125]I-ME 491 bound directly to DNA or to a specific nonhistone chromatin proteins. *Hinc*II-digested chromatin of SW948 colorectal carcinoma cells was immunoprecipitated (Figure 9) with mAb ME 491.[79] A 55,000-$M_r$ single chromatin protein was specifically immunoprecipitated by mAb ME 491, but not by any other mAb tested. Thus nuclear antigen for mAb ME 491 exhibits a molecular weight different[79] than the cell surface antigen ME 491 ($M_r$ 30 to 60,000).[90]

The aim of experiment 3 was to determine whether mAb ME 491 was randomly distributed in the chromatin or instead bound to a specific chromatin region. Chromatin was isolated from cells exposed for 24 h to [125]I-mAb 491 (100 ng/ml), and digested with *Bam*HI or *Hinc*II.[79] Restriction nuclease-digested chromatin contains the ternary complexes which represent a mixture of DNA fragments attached to chromatin proteins; they consist of DNA fragment(s)-ME 491 chromatin antigen-[125]I-mAb ME 491 and may be electrophoretically separated.[79] If the electrophoresis is performed in non-dissociating and non-reducing conditions, the ternary complexes are intact and may be autoradiographically detected in the gel.[78,79] In the case of [125]I-mAb ME 491 bound to the chromatin of colorectal carcinoma cells, *Bam*HI did not release any ternary complexes, while sequential digestion with *Hinc*II released two ternary complexes, one of the lower and one of the higher molecular weight (Figure 10). The results obtained suggest that the [125]I-mAb 491 binds to very specific fragments of chromatin.

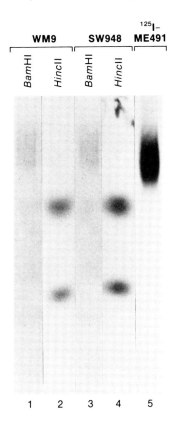

**FIGURE 10.** Electrophoretic analysis and autoradiographic detection (4% polyacrylamide gel) of restriction nuclease-digested chromatin isolated from cells incubated with [125]I-mAb ME 491 for 24 h. After a 24 h digestion with *Bam*HI, the remaining chromatin was digested with *Hinc*II for 24 h. (From Rakowicz-Szulczynska, E. and Koprowski, H., *Arch. Biochem. Biophys.*, 271, 366, 1989. With permission.)

*Nuclear translocation of mAb ME 491 in a cell-free system* — In order to check whether mAb ME 491 is able to enter the isolated nucleus in the absence of the cell surface antigen or instead requires ME 491 or another vehicle protein, experiments were performed in a cell-free system.[79] After exposure of the isolated nuclei to [125]I-mAb ME 491 in the synthetic medium, the nondegraded mAb was found inside the nucleus, tightly bound to the chromatin (Figure 11). Thus, mAb ME 491 requires neither the ME 491 antigen nor a cytoplasmic protein to enter the nucleus.

mAb ME 491 did not immunoprecipitate any protein from the nuclear membrane fraction (not shown), which suggests that translocation across the nuclear membrane occurs through the different mechanism than that which may involve mAb ME 491-recognized nuclear membrane-associated antigen.

To test whether mAb ME 491 is translocated across the nuclear membrane through the mediation of the nuclear pore receptor which contains N-acetylamide

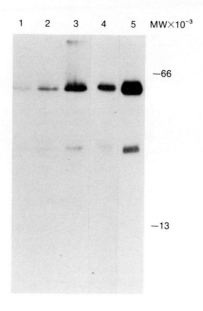

**FIGURE 11.** Autoradiogram of SDS-PAGE (10% polyacrylamide gel) of [125]I-mAb ME 491 incorporated into the chromatin of SW948 colorectal carcinoma cell nuclei incubated for 2 h at room temperature with [125]I-mAb ME 491 in crude cytoplasm (lane 1), membrane-free cytosol (lane 2), or incubation medium (lane 3). [125]I-mAb ME 491 remaining in the crude cytoplasm after 2 h incubation with nuclei (lane 4); free [125]I-mAb ME 491 used in experiment (lane 5). (From Rakowicz-Szulczynska, E. and Koprowski, H., *Arch. Biochem. Biophys.*, 271, 366, 1989. With permission.)

galactosamine and is sensitive to WGA treatment,[111,112] nuclear translocation of mAb ME 491 in the presence or absence of WGA was compared (Table 6). It was surprising to find that treatment of the nuclei with WGA significantly activated (more than threefold) mAb ME 491 translocation to the nucleus. The results suggest that at least the major part of mAb ME 491 is not translocated to the nucleus through the classical mechanism of interaction of the signal sequences containing protein with the nuclear pore receptor.[94,95] Instead, blocking of that receptor by the lectin (WGA) seems to activate another mechanism(s) of mAb translocation to the nucleus. The described activatory effect of WGA on nuclear translocation of mAb ME 491 is unique and was not detected in the case of the other mAb tested. Since mAb ME 491 is of the isotype IgM, while other mAb tested are IgG, we can suggest that different mechanisms of nuclear translocation for different mAb may exist.

Nuclear translocation of mAb ME 491 was specific; at the same conditions, the mAb Br15-6A against carbohydrate Y determinant expressed by cancer cells did not enter the nuclei. Nuclear uptake of a protein (BSA, 66,000) of lower molecular weight than IgM was also tested as a control for the possibility of a passive diffusion of mAb ME 491 through the nuclear membrane. [125]I-BSA showed no nuclear translocation in any of the experiments.[79] Other low-molecular-weight proteins like EGF (6000) and IGF-I (7000) were also not incorporated into the isolated nuclei which eliminates nuclear damage during the experiment and passive uptake of mAb ME 491. Although [125]I-mAb ME 491 was effectively translocated into the nuclei (Table 6) resuspended in the chemically-defined mechanism, the presence of a cytoplasmic protein regulating or activating nuclear translocation of this mAb *in vivo* could not be eliminated.

To determine whether any cytoplasmic component might be potentially involved in nuclear translocation of mAb ME 491, isolated nuclei were incubated in the presence of crude (membrane-containing) cytoplasm, pure (membrane-free) cytosol, or the chemically defined medium mixed with microsomal at fraction[79] (Table 7). Instead of the expected activation of the nuclear translocation of the [125]I-mAb ME 491 in the presence of the cell membrane antigen-containing microsomal fraction, uptake of the mAb ME 491 in the presence of microsomal fraction added to the synthetic medium was reduced to 86% of the level of nuclear translocation occurring in the incubation medium alone, compared to 75% the level of nuclear uptake of mAb ME 491 in the crude cytoplasm, and 12.5% in the presence of the membrane-free cytosol. The results obtained strongly suggest that nuclear translocation of mAb ME 491 does not require binding to the cell surface antigen or to any other cytoplasmic protein. Instead, present in the cytoplasm or the microsomal fraction, protein(s) or other components must bind mAb ME 491 and inhibit competitively nuclear uptake of mAb ME 491.

When the cytosol was isolated from cells that were exposed to mAb ME 491 (12 h, 100 mg/ml) nuclear uptake of mAb ME 491 was only slightly lower than that occurring in the synthesis medium (Table 7). The last result suggests that in intact cells, mAb ME 491 saturated the pool of ME 491 antigen, which, after isolation of the cytoplasm, did not block the mAb ME 491 entry in the nucleus.

To verify the above hypothesis and identify the cytoplasmic component competing for mAb ME 491 in nuclear transport, the cytoplasmic fraction was isolated from cells labeled with [[35]S]methionine and [[35]S]cysteine, centrifuged to remove the microsomal fraction, and incubated with mAb ME 491.[79] A precipitate was formed, which was analyzed electrophoretically in a 10% gel with SDS under reducing conditions. Two proteins of 190,000 $M_r$ and 42,000 $M_r$ were detected at the autoradiogram (Figure 12A). The 42-kDa protein was not observed when the cytoplasm was first chromatographed on a Sepharose CL4B-protein A-anti-actin IgG column; thus it represents cytoplasmic actin.

To determine whether the 190-kDa band represents a cytoplasmic protein alone or a complex containing mAb ME 491, the unlabeled cytosol was incubated with [125]I-mAb ME 491 in the presence of a crosslinking agent (dimethyl suberimidate).[79] A 190-kDa band, containing cross-linked [125]I-mAb ME 491, was again observed (Figure 12B). Since the molecular weight of ME 491 antigen predicted on the basis of cDNA is 25,000,[76] we may suggest that mAb ME 491 binds to two ME 491 antigen molecules synthesized and present in the cytoplasm and that the complex resists dissociation by SDS. Alternatively, mAb ME 491 may bind to the 55 kDa chromatin antigen, which also must be synthesized in the cytoplasm. The ME 491 antigens detected by mAb ME 491 in the membrane-free cytosol could represent a free antigen as well as being bound to a polysomal complex (the antigen which just was being synthesized). To test the last possibility, the precipitate was analyzed

## TABLE 7
### Effect of the Cytoplasmic and Plasma Membrane Proteins on Nuclear Translocation of $^{125}$I-mAb ME 491 in a Cell-Free System

| | | | Chromatin-bound molecules per nucleus[a] | | | | | |
|---|---|---|---|---|---|---|---|---|
| Cell line | Incubation medium | %[b] | Incubation medium plus microsomal fraction | %[b] | Crude cytoplasm | %[b] | Pure cytosol | %[b] |
| WM9 | 10,000 | 100 | 8,600 | 86 | 750 | 7.5 | 1,250 | 12.5 |
| | | | | | | | 8,200[c] | 82 |
| SW948 | 14,200 | 100 | 12,000 | 84.5 | 2,450 | 17.2 | 5,100 | 35 |
| | | | | | | | 12,300[c] | 86.6 |

[a]  Data are given as means from three experiments; SD = 12%.
[b]  Data are shown as percentage of the nucleus uptake, where uptake in the incubation medium (0.25 $M$ sucrose, 20 m$M$ Tris-HCl, pH 7.8, 10 m$M$ MgCl$_2$, 500 ng/ml BSA).
[c]  Cytosol was isolated from cells preincubated 12 h with mAb ME 491 (100 ng/ml).

for the presence of ME 491 antigen mRNA, which would be expected to precipitate together with the protein.[79] RNA isolated from the precipitate was separated in agarose gels containing formaldehyde, transferred to nitrocellulose, and analyzed by Northern blot hybridization with a [$^{32}$P]TTP-labeled cDNA probe for the ME 491 antigen. Strong hybridization signals were detected (Figure 13), which suggests that mRNA for ME 491 antigen was coprecipitated by mAb ME 491.[79] To further test specificity of precipitation, we have tested the presence of α-enolase mRNA in the precipitate containing mRNA for the ME 491 antigen. The control cDNA probe for α-enolase showed no hybridization with RNA of the precipitate. Thus, we concluded that mAb ME 491 binds to the newly synthesized antigen ME 491 and specifically precipitates polysomal mRNA of this antigen from the cytoplasm.[79]

To analyze whether the polysomal interaction of mAb ME 491 with the synthesized antigen represents an artifact observed after cell fractionation, or instead $^{125}$I-mAb ME 491 internalized into the cytoplasm of intact cells also interacts with the newly synthesized ME 491 antigen, an effect of the polysomal complex on the transport of $^{125}$I-mAb ME 491 to the nucleus was tested. The intracellular level of the ME 491-containing polysomal complexes was modulated by cell preincubation with inhibitors of protein biosynthesis[79] (Table 8). Preincubation of cells for 1 h with puromycin, which prematurely releases mRNA from the ribosomes, inhibited protein biosynthesis by 85%, and resulted in an increase in nuclear uptake and chromatin binding of mAb ME 491 to 43% of total internalized mAb, compared to 5% of chromatin-bound mAb ME 491 in cells not exposed to puromycin. Redistribution of $^{125}$I-mAb ME 491 occurred without changes in total intracellular uptake and chromatin binding of $^{125}$I-mAb ME 491.[79] With actinomycin D, which inhibits RNA transcription, protein synthesis decreased after 1 h by 65%, while the nuclear uptake and chromatin binding of $^{125}$I-mAb ME 491 increased to 51% (Table 8).[79] An increase in nuclear uptake of mAb ME 491 after inhibition of protein synthesis that occurred without a change in total intracellular uptake suggested that a protein(s)

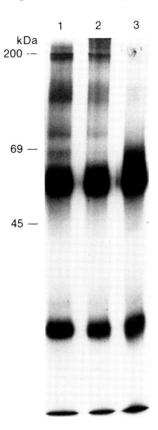

**FIGURE 12.**  Autoradiogram of SDS-PAGE (5% polyacrylamide gel) of the precipitate formed after incubation of [125]I-mAb ME 491 (0.01 μg) with unlabeled cytosol from SW948 cells, in the presence of cross-linking agent (dimethyl suberimidate) and in the absence (lanes 1 and 2) or presence of unlabeled mAb ME 491 (2 μg) (lane 3). The protein bands of the $M_r$ 200,000 (lanes 1 and 2) represent mAb ME 491 cross-linked to the synthesized antigen ME 491. Binding of the [125]I-mAb ME 491 (lanes 1 and 2) is competitively blocked by the excess of unlabeled mAb ME 491 (lane 3). Strong radioactive bands of heavy and light chain chains of [125]I-mAb ME 491 are also visible (lanes 1 to 3). (From Rakowicz-Szulczynska, E. and Koprowski, H., *Arch. Biochem. Biophys.*, 271, 366, 1989. With permission.)

synthesized in the cytoplasm may block the nuclear uptake of mAb ME 491. Since in a cell-free system, [125]I-mAb ME 491 binds to the newly synthesized ME 491 antigen(s), we suggest that *in vivo* a fraction of the mAb ME 491 internalized and released from the lysosomal membranes binds to the synthesized antigen(s).

Exactly how the ME 491 antigen, which like all membrane proteins must be translocated into the lumen during synthesis, interacts with internalized by the cell mAb ME 491 also remains unclear. However, the interaction occurs efficiently in

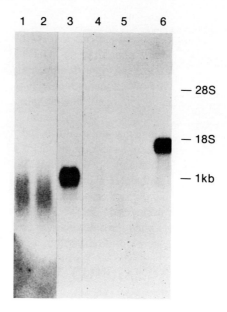

**FIGURE 13.** Northern blot hybridization of RNA precipitated with mAb ME 491 from WM9 melanoma (lanes 1 and 4) and SW948 colorectal carcinoma (lanes 2 and 5) cell cytoplasm and of control RNA from ME 491 antigen-expressing cells (lanes 3 and 6) with [$^{32}$P]-labeled DNA probe for ME 491 gene (lanes 1 to 3) and for α-enolase gene (lanes 4 to 6). Lanes 4 to 6 represent the same filter as lanes 1 to 3 which was dehybridized and hybridized with the control probe (α-enolase gene). (From Rakowicz-Szulczynska, E. and Koprowski, H., *Arch. Biochem. Biophys.*, 271, 366, 1989. With permission.)

## TABLE 8
### Chromatin Binding of $^{125}$I-mAb ME 491 in Intact WM9 Cells after 1 or 3 h Preincubation with Inhibitors of Protein Biosynthesis Followed by a 1-h Exposure to $^{125}$I-mAb ME 491

| Preincubation | Total uptake (molecules per cell[a]) | | Chromatin binding (%) | | Protein synthesis[b] (%) | |
|---|---|---|---|---|---|---|
| | 1 h[c] | 3 h[c] | 1 h | 3 h | 1 h | 3 h |
| Culture medium | 10,000 | 10,000 | 5 | 5.5 | 100 | 100 |
| Puromycin (200 μg/ml) | 10,500 | 980 | 43 | 3.8 | 15 | 5 |
| Actinomycin D | 10,800 | 1,200 | 51 | 4 | 35 | 20 |

[a]   The mean from three experiments; SD exceeded 10 to 15%.
[b]   Protein synthesis was measured as [$^{35}$S]methionine incorporation into 10% TCA-precipitable fraction of the cell lysate in 10 m$M$ Tris-HCL, pH 7, 1 m$M$ PMSF.
[c]   Times of preincubation.

a cell-free system after centrifugation of the membranes. Even under hypotonic conditions, it seems unlikely that newly synthesized ME 491 is released from the lumen instead of being covered by vesicles pinched off from the endoplasmic reticulum. Presence of the *de novo* synthesized cell surface antigen in the membrane-free cytosol represents a general phenomenon. It is likely that two types of antigens are expressed, one membrane-bound and delivered to the cell membrane (surface) and another type of the free cytosolic antigens. Association of the antigen with the polysomal complex and its presence in the membrane-free cytosol allows detection and purification of both antigen and the corresponding mRNA by ligand (growth factor or mAb) precipitation.[113] The role of the internalized ligand association with the antigen-mRNA complex remains unknown. It is likely that such interaction may have a critical role in regulation of the amount of the ligand translocated to the nucleus and/or the number of receptors expressed on the cell surface, mRNA stability, etc.

*Effect of mAb ME 491 on transcription* — To determine whether nuclear translocation of mAb ME 491 has any effect on transcription, RNA synthesis in intact SW948 cells was measured after 1 or 24 h exposure to mAb ME 491 and after 1 h of exposure of nuclei isolated from the same cells (Table 9). In intact cells exposed to 100 ng/ml mAb ME 491, total RNA synthesis, measured as [³H]uridine incorporation into cytoplasmic, nucleoplasmic, and chromatin RNA, decreased by 74% after 1 h[79] (Table 9, Experiment A). To determine whether mAb ME 491 taken up by the nucleus directly affects transcription, RNA synthesis was tested in isolated nuclei. After a 1-h exposure to mAb ME 491 at 10 ng/ml, RNA synthesis in isolated nuclei, measured as incorporation of [³²P]UTP, decreased by 55%. Higher concentrations of mAb ME 491 affected RNA synthesis by 60% (not shown). Thus mAb ME 491 taken up by the nucleus and bound to chromatin may directly inhibit transcription. Since ribosomal RNA represents the bulk of synthesized RNA, we analyzed the effect of mAb ME 491 taken up by the nucleus on rRNA synthesis. [³²P]UTP RNA synthesized in SW948 cell nuclei in the presence or absence of mAb ME 491 was hybridized to plasmid DNA containing the ribosomal DNA. Transcription levels of rRNA in nuclei incubated with mAb ME 491 decreased by 67% as compared with transcription levels in nuclei of control cells (Table 9). Thus, mAb ME 491 taken up by nucleus and bound to chromatin directly inhibited transcription of ribosomal RNA genes.[79]

*mAb ME 491 as an artificial ligand for a growth factor receptor* — Three targets may be distinguished in mAb ME 491 interaction with the cell: cell surface ME 491 antigen, synthesized on the polysoma ME 491 antigen(s), and nuclear antigen p55. The intracellular action of mAb ME 491 resembles the interaction of growth factors with the newly synthesized receptor and with the chromatin receptor. The hypothetical model of mAb ME 491 action is summarized in Figure 14. mAb ME 491 enters the cell through the mediation of the cell surface ME 491 antigen. When inside the cell, a fraction of mAb ME 491 molecules interact with the synthesized, polysomes-bound ME 491 antigen, while another fraction of mAb ME 491 penetrates the nucleus and binds to the chromatin. Binding of mAb ME 491

## TABLE 9
### Incorporation of [³H]Uridine into Intact SW948 Cells Incubated 1 h with mAb ME 491 (Experiment A) and of [³²P]UTP into Isolated Nuclei Incubated 1 h with mAb ME 491 (Experiment B)

| mAb ME 491 (ng/ml) | Experiment A Incorporation (cpm per 10⁶ cells) of [³H]Uridine into cellular RNA[a] | % total RNA synthesis inhibition | Experiment B Incorporation (cpm per 10⁶ cells) of [³²P]UTP into nuclear RNA[a] | % total RNA synthesis inhibition | [³²P]UTP hybridization to rDNA[b] cpm | % inhibition |
|---|---|---|---|---|---|---|
| 0 | 37,500 | 0 | 62,000 | 0 | 24,100 | 0 |
| 100 | 10,000 | 74 | 28,000 | 55 | 8,000 | 67 |

[a]  Mean from four experiments (SD = 10 to 15%).
[b]  Mean from two experiments (SD = 5%).

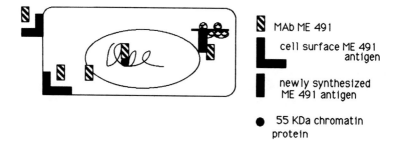

**FIGURE 14.**    Hypothetical model of mAb ME 491 action. mAb ME 491 taken up through the mediation of the cell surface ME 491 antigen is released in the cytoplasm. Some of the mAb ME 491 molecules in the cytoplasm interact with the newly synthesized ME 491 antigen while other molecules penetrate the nucleus and bind to the chromatin 55-kDa protein. Binding of mAb ME 491 to the chromatin 55-kDa protein inhibits transcription of ribosomal DNA. (From Rakowicz-Szulczynska, E. and Koprowski, H., *Arch. Biochem. Biophys.*, 271, 366, 1989. With permission.)

occurs to specific chromatin regions and is likely to be mediated by the antigen p55. Interaction of mAb ME 491 with the chromatin results in inhibition of rRNA synthesis.[79] The inhibitory effect of mAb ME 491 on synthesis of rRNA is quantitatively very similar to the effected mediated by NGF.[109] We postulate that mAb ME 491 which is directed against the cell surface glycoprotein (ME 491) may mimic an intracellular pathway of yet unknown ligand, recognized by the same ME 491 antigen. The chromatin-bound 55,000-$M_r$ protein immunoprecipitated by mAb ME 491 may represent the original nuclear receptor for that unknown ligand.

The conserved function of some molecules may be brought to light by studies of conformational or structural homology of antigenic epitopes expressed by the evolutionarily unrelated organisms. Sequence analysis suggests that tumor-associated antigen ME 491,[90] colon carcinoma associated antigen CO-029,[114] the leukocyte cell surface antigens CD37,[115] CD9,[116] CD53,[117] TAPA-1,[118] and the Sm23 antigen of the parasitic helminth *Schistosoma mansoni*[119] belong to a common family of cell surface antigens.[114] The newest studies indicate antigenic identity of ME 491, with another melanoma antigen NK1/C-3 and neuroglandular antigen.[120] Since mAb ME 491 is internalized by cells and translocated to the cell nucleus and inhibits transcription of ribosomal RNA,[79] it is likely that the original ligand recognized by ME 491 antigen is involved in regulation of cell growth. The evolutionary conservation of that antigen supports that hypothesis. Therefore, although the original ligand recognized by ME 491 is unknown, it may be suggested that if such a ligand exists it may activate or inhibit rRNA synthesis and thereby affect cell growth. If the hypothetical ligand acts as a stimulator of rRNA synthesis, then mAb ME 491 antagonizes that effect. The hypothetical ligand to ME 491 antigen, which is able to activate rRNA synthesis, would exhibit similar effects as the fibroblast growth factor[121] and platelet-derived growth factor,[110] both of which localize in the nucleus and activate rRNA synthesis. If the original ligand represents an inhibitor of rRNA synthesis, it would act similarly to NGF.[109,110] Since increased or decreased rRNA levels activate or inhibit, respectively, protein synthesis and thereby cell growth, the original ligand to ME 491 may play an important role in regulation of cell growth. In that case mAb ME 491 may replace and act as antagonist of the original ligands. Theoretically ME 491 would be used as a carrier of a toxin or as a radioactive ligand. Since antigen ME 491 is expressed not only on tumors, but also on normal cells, the interesting mechanism of its action is unlikely to be useful in therapy of human tumors.

## C. MONOCLONAL ANTIBODIES DIRECTED TO THE CARBOHYDRATE DETERMINANTS EXPRESSED ON THE TUMOR CELL SURFACE

The binding domains of most known mAb against carbohydrate antigens include the terminal saccharide chains of glycolipids and glycoproteins.[122,123] Most of the sugar epitopes expressed on tumor cells involve galactose/galactosamine, fucose, and neuraminic acid. Interaction of antibodies with the carbohydrate epitope was mainly studied using synthetic carbohydrate determinants.[123,124] Since the same carbohydrate determinant may be expressed by different glycoproteins as well as by glycolipids, it is likely that the effect raised by the mAb against a carbohydrate epitope would be varied, depending on the core proteins attached to this epitope. Our experiments with different mAb able to recognize carbohydrate domains (Table 1) indicated that only one mAb against the carbohydrate Y determinant is internalized, while none of the other mAb tested (against Lewis[a], Lewis[b], GD2/GD3) enters the cell. The mechanism of anti-carbohydrate mAb (mAb Br 15-6A) internalization was tested.[80]

### 1. Intracellular Localization of mAb Br 15-6A by Immunofluorescence Staining

mAb Br 15-1A (IgG2a) is directed against the carbohydrate Y determinant and expressed on tumor but not on normal cells.[99] Another mAb tested, mAb Br 55.2

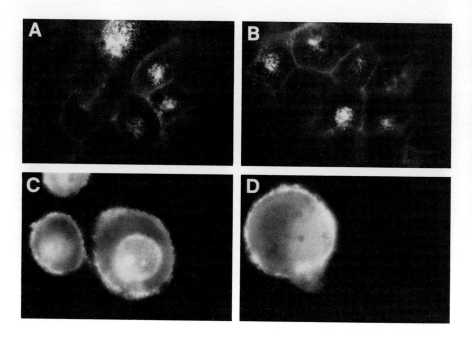

**FIGURE 15.** Immunofluorescence staining of SW1116 cells (A), SW707 cells (B), and SKBr 5 cells (C, D) incubated for 18 h with mAb Br 15-6A (300 ng/ml) (A to C) or with mAb Br 55.2 (300 ng/ml) (D) with fluoresceine-conjugated sheep anti-mouse IgG. Nuclei were stained positively after incubation of SW707 cells with NGF (10 ng/ml), followed by rabbit to NGF serum and fluoresceine-conjugated goat anti-rabbit IgG (E). Nuclei were stained negatively when mAb Br 15-6A was bound to colloidal gold (F). As a control, SW707 cells were incubated with fluoresceine-conjugated anti-mouse IgG (G). (From Rakowicz-Szulczynska, E., Steplewski, Z., and Koprowski, H., *Am. J. Pathology,* 141, 937, 1992. With permission.)

(IgG2a, IgG3), recognizes the Y determinant and the B structure as well.[99] The Y determinant is expressed as glycolipid or glycoprotein. Association of Y with the EGF receptor was also described.[100]

After 24 h of incubation of SW1116, SW707 colorectal carcinoma cells, and SKBr 5 breast carcinoma cells with mAb Br 15-6A, followed by incubation with fluoresceine-conjugated goat anti-mouse IgG, fluorescence was detected inside the cell[80] (Figure 15A-C). In contrast to mAb Br 15-6A, mAb Br 55.2 bound to the cell surface but did not penetrate the cells, as indicated by the fluorescence ring surrounding the cells (Figure 15D). In SKBr 5 cells, fluorescence of mAb Br 15.6A in the nuclei was stronger than that of the cytoplasm, and the shape of the nucleus was well visible (Figure 15C). In SW1116 (Figure 15A) and SW707 (Figure 15B) cells, which incorporate less mAb Br 15-6A molecules, the shape of the nucleus was not visible, and it is difficult to determine whether mAb Br 15-6A localized to the nucleus or to the Golgi apparatus. Nonspecific adsorption of the sheep anti-mouse IgG to human cells may be eliminated, since cells not preincubated with mAb Br 15-6A or mAb Br 55.2 showed negative staining (not shown). Comparing

## TABLE 10
## Intracellular Distribution of $^{125}$I-mAb Br 15-6A, $^{125}$I-mAb Br 55.2 and $^{125}$I-mAb 425 after 4 h Incubation with Different Tumor Cell Lines

| Cell line | Cell or cell fraction[b] | Molecules per cell[a] | | | | |
|---|---|---|---|---|---|---|
| | | $^{125}$I-mAb Br 15-6A | | $^{125}$I-mAb Br 55.2 | $^{125}$I-mAb 425 | |
| SKBr 5 | Cell | 250,000 | | 300,000 | 35,000 | |
| | C | 175,840 | | <300 | 20,620 | |
| | N | 3,520 | CH/C[c] | 10 | 9 | CH/C |
| | NM | 7,540 | 0.16 | 5 | 1 | 0.02 |
| | CH | 27,535 | | 5 | 400 | |
| SW1116 | Cell | 30,500 | | 35,800 | 22,500 | |
| | C | 17,750 | | 200 | 15,100 | |
| | N | 1,100 | CH/C | 10 | 500 | CH/C |
| | NM | 1,400 | 0.17 | 0 | 125 | 0.01 |
| | CH | 3,050 | | 5 | 275 | |
| SW707 | Cell | 24,000 | | 28,000 | 890 | |
| | C | 7,000 | | 200 | | |
| | N | 2,200 | CH/C | 0 | <400 | |
| | NM | 750 | 0.14 | 0 | | |
| | CH | 1,000 | | 5 | | |
| SW948 | Cell | 6,050 | | 6,900 | 70,000 | |
| | C | | | | 40,500 | |
| | N | <200 | | <150 | 500 | CH/C |
| | NM | | | | 800 | 0.05 |
| | CH | | | | 1,900 | |
| A431 | Cell | Not tested | | Not tested | Not tested | |
| | C | | | | 360,790 | |
| | N | <100 | | <80 | 4,500 | CH/C |
| | NM | | | | 1,200 | 0.04 |
| | CH | | | | 14,000 | |
| V87 Mg | Cell | Not tested | | Not tested | 84,000 | |
| | C | | | | 68,500 | |
| | N | <120 | | <100 | 180 | CH/C |
| | NM | | | | 250 | 0.02 |
| | CH | | | | 1,300 | |

[a]   Mean from five experiments; SD = 5% for chromatin and 12% for other fractions.
[b]   C = membrane-free cytoplasm; N = nucleoplasm; NM = nuclear membrane; CH = chromatin.
[c]   CH/C is the ratio between the number of mAb molecules encountered in the chromatin and in the cytoplasm.

From Rakowicz-Szulczynska, E., Steplewski, Z., and Koprowski, H., *Am. J. Pathology*, 141, 937, 1992. With permission.

the distribution of mAb Br 15-6A fluorescence inside the cells with those of mAb directed against breast cancer cells (Figure 4) or mAb ME 491 (Figure 7), we have concluded that distribution of each mAb inside the cell and inside the nucleus is highly specific.

## 2. Internalization and Chromatin Binding of $^{125}$I-mAb Br 15-6A

Since the Y determinant recognized by mAb Br 15-6A is expressed by EGF receptor as well as by other proteins, we suspected that mAb Br 15-1A may be internalized by EGF receptor which mediates internalization of EGF and mAb 425 (see Section A). To test this possibility, we compared internalization of $^{125}$I-mAb Br 15-1A with internalization of $^{125}$I-mAb 425 directed against protein domain of the EGF receptor (Table 10). The experiments eliminated correlation between mAb 425 and mAb Br 15-6A uptake. $^{125}$I-mAb Br 15-6A was bound to the cell surface of A431 epidermoid carcinoma; SKBr 5 breast carcinoma; SW1116, SW707, and SW948 colorectal carcinoma; and glioma V 373 cell lines. In the breast carcinoma SKBr 5 and in SW1116 and SW707 colorectal carcinoma cell lines, the mAb was internalized and taken up by the nucleus.[80] Cells of epidermoid carcinoma A 431, which express a high number of cell surface EGF receptors, internalized the highest number of mAb 425 molecules, but did not show internalization of the mAb Br 15-6A. Cells of colorectal carcinoma SW948, which express EGF receptor,[78] also did not internalize Br 15-6A but did internalize mAb 425. In contrast, SW707 colorectal carcinoma cells, which show a very low level of the EGF receptors,[78] did not internalize mAb 425, but did internalize mAb Br 15-6A. Only cells of SKBr 5 breast carcinoma and SW1116 colorectal carcinoma internalized both mAb Br 15-6A and mAb 425. Breast carcinoma cells internalized a higher number of mAb Br 15-6A molecules than of mAb 425. These results may, however, reflect lower numbers of mAb 425 molecules to the surface of SKBr5 cells.

$^{125}$I-mAb Br 55.2, which also binds to Y and B determinants, bound to the cell surface of the tested cell lines in slightly higher amounts than $^{125}$I-mAb Br 15-6A, but did not internalize (Table 11), which confirms the negative staining of the nucleus and cytoplasm in the immunofluorescence staining (Figure 14D). A selective internalization of mAb Br 15-6A, but not of mAb Br 55.2, eliminates the possibility of nonspecific adsorption of $^{125}$I-IgG to cell organelles during fractionation. It also indicates that binding of mAb Br 55.2 to the cell surface is not sufficient for internalization of these mAb.[80]

Lack of correlation between mAb 425 and mAb Br 15-1A internalization eliminates the role of EGF receptor in internalization of mAb Br 15-1A. Internalization of mAb Br 15-6A was blocked in 98% at 0°C, which proves that mAb Br 15-6A was taken up through the active process, probably through the mediation of a molecule different from the EGF receptor. Since a fraction of internalized mAb Br 15-6A localized to the cell nucleus and was bound to the chromatin, it was likely that chromatin also expresses an antigen recognized by mAb Br 15-6A.

## 3. Immunoprecipitation of the Cell Surface and the Chromatin Antigens Recognized by mAb Br 15-6A

To determine whether mAb Br 15-6A is specifically internalized through a Y-determinant-associated cell surface protein, extracts of cytoplasmic membranes (prepared from cells of SKBr 5, SW1116, and SW707 lines) were immunoprecipitated with both mAb Br 15-6A and mAb Br 55.2.[80] mAb Br 55.2, which is not internalized, was used to eliminate the possibility that mAb Br 15-6A binds to a protein that does not express the Y determinant recognized by both mAb. Both mAb Br 15-6A and mAb Br 55.2 immunoprecipitated a 108,000 $M_r$ molecule from the membranes of the colorectal carcinoma cells (Figure 16; lanes 1 to 4) and a 92,000 to 96,000 $M_r$ protein from the membranes of breast carcinoma cells (lanes 9, 11). The 108,000 $M_r$ protein was not precipitated by control mAb P3 (not shown). Several low molecular weight proteins were coprecipitated by mAb Br 15-6A and mAb Br 55.2 from the membrane fractions. Since the Y determinant is attached to several proteins, it is likely that both mAb immunoprecipitated a whole family of Y-associated proteins. We cannot, however, eliminate the possibility that some of these proteins may originate in the process of degradation of the 108,000 or 92,000 to 96,000 $M_r$ proteins. By increasing salt concentrations during immunoprecipitation (from 0.14 $M$ NaCl to 0.25 $M$ NaCl), we were able to eliminate several low molecular protein bands[80] (not shown), which further indicates that the 108,000 $M_r$ protein in colorectal carcinoma cells represents the antigen which binds mAb Br 15-6A with highest affinity. No protein was specifically immunoprecipitated from V87 Mg glioma cells (Figure 16; lanes 14, 15).

Since glioma cells do not express a 108,000 $M_r$ or 92,000 to 96,000 $M_r$ proteins and do not internalize mAb Br 15-6A, we suggest that these proteins may be somehow involved in internalization of mAb Br 15-6A.

To establish further whether mAb Br 15-6A which is internalized and translocated to the nucleus binds to a specific chromatin protein, chromatin was isolated from different tumor cell lines labeled with [$^{35}$S]methionine, digested with *Eco*RI and immunoprecipitated with mAb Br 15-6A and mAb Br 55.2 (Figure 16).

Both mAb Br 15-6A and mAb Br 55.2 immunoprecipitated an 88,000 $M_r$ antigen from the chromatin of colorectal SW707[80] (Figure 16; lanes 5, 7), SW1116 (not shown), and breast carcinoma SKBr 5 (Figure 16; lanes 8, 10). Immunoprecipitation with mAb Br 15-6A of the chromatin fraction remaining after immunoprecipitation with mAb Br 55.2 did not reveal any protein (not shown). Thus, both mAb Br 15-6A and mAb Br 55.2 bind to the same antigen. The 88,000 $M_r$ protein was not immunoprecipitated with nonspecific mAb P3 (Figure 16; lane 6). The 88,000 $M_r$ chromatin protein was also not recognized by mAb 425 (not shown). In addition to 88,000 $M_r$ proteins, several low molecular weight chromatin proteins coimmunoprecipitated. Since we immunoprecipitate DNA-protein complexes obtained after chromatin digestion with a restriction nuclease, it is likely that several proteins bound to the same restriction fragment may precipitate together with 88,000 $M_r$ proteins. This suggestion is supported by the fact that increased salt concentration did not eliminate these proteins[80] (not shown). However, we cannot eliminate the possibility that in addition to the 88,000 $M_r$ protein, another low molecular weight protein(s) is involved in binding mAb Br 15-6A.

To determine whether the cell surface and the chromatin proteins that are immunoprecipitated by mAb Br 15-6A are localized in two different cellular compartments, and to eliminate a possibility that the chromatin protein is a degradation product of the cell surface antigen that attaches to the nucleus during preparation,

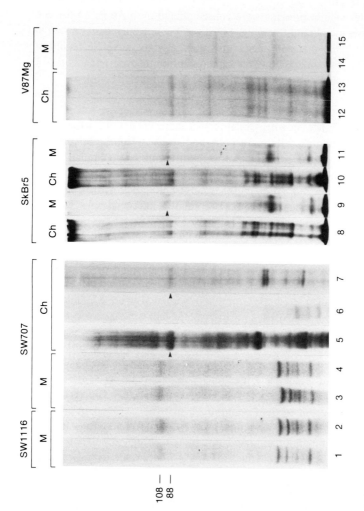

108 —
88 —

**FIGURE 16.** Autoradiograms of SDS-polyacrylamide gel electrophoresis (7.5% polyacrylamide gel) of proteins immunoprecipitated by mAb Br 15-6A or mAb Br 55.2 from membranes (M) and from *Eco*RI-digested chromatin (Ch) (2 × 10⁷ cells). The 108,000-$M_r$ protein was immunoprecipitated from membranes of SW1116 and SW707 colorectal carcinoma cells with mAb Br 15-6A (lanes 1 and 3) or with mAb Br 55.2 (lanes 2 and 4) and the 92,000 to 96,000 $M_r$ protein from membranes of SKBr 5 breast carcinoma cells (lane 9, mAb Br 15-6A; lane 11, mAb Br 55.2). Neither 108,000 $M_r$, nor 92,000 to 96,000 $M_r$, proteins were detected by mAb Br 15-6A (lane 14) or mAb Br 55.2 (lane 15) in V87Mg glioma cells. The 88,000 $M_r$, protein was immunoprecipitated from the chromatin of all cell lines by both mAb Br 15-6A (lanes 7 and 12) or mAb Br 55.2 (lanes 5, 10, and 13). Nonspecific mAb P3 (lane 6) did not immunoprecipitate any high molecular weight chromatin protein. Autoradiographic detection of [³⁵S]methionine-labeled proteins after 2 d of exposure.

the inner nuclear membrane and the nucleoplasm (which remain on the top of 1.7 *M* sucrose used for purification of the chromatin) were immunoprecipitated with both mAb. No protein was specifically immunoprecipitated by mAb Br 15-6A from nuclear membranes or from nucleoplasm (not shown), which suggests that the isolated nuclei are free of cell membrane contamination. Since both cell surface and chromatic antigens were immunoprecipitated from cells not exposed to mAb Br 15-6A, it is likely that mAb Br 15-6A (and also mAb 55.2) recognize two antigens localized in different cell compartments.

Since both mAb Br 15-6A and mAb Br 55.2 recognized the same cell surface antigen, and moreover, both mAb detected the same nuclear antigen (Figure 15), it seems that internalization of mAb Br 15-6A is dependent on the very specific stereochemical interaction of the mAb with the Y-associated cell surface protein (Figure 16). The Y determinant represents probably only a part of the epitope recognized by both mAb, while the other part of the epitope must be represented by protein domain. The same protein is recognized by mAb Br 55.2, but different stereochemical interaction is likely to block the internalization. Thus, binding of a ligand to an internalizable antigen is not sufficient to induce the process of internalization.

The cell-free system experiments indicated that neither mAb Br 15-6A nor Br 55.2 are taken up by isolated nuclei (not shown). These results suggest that *in vivo* nuclear translocation of the mAb Br 15-6A internalized into the cytoplasm requires a prior activation by binding to the cell surface receptor or to a cytoplasmic protein, which mediates nuclear entry. It further confirms the hypothesis that different intracellular mechanisms regulate nuclear translocation of particular antibodies.

## 4. Specificity of the Chromatin Binding of mAb Br 15-6A

Electrophoretic analysis of the $^{125}$I-mAb Br 15-6A extracted from the chromatin showed that the $M_r$ of both light and heavy chains of this mAb were the same as of the native IgG, which suggests that mAb Br 15-6A was taken up by the nucleus in nondegraded form[80] (Figure 17).

To establish whether mAb Br 15-6A binds to specific chromatin regions or is randomly distributed, chromatin isolated from SW1116, SW707, and SKBr 5 (incubated with $^{125}$I-Br 15-6A) was digested with three different restriction enzymes: *Eco*RI, *Hinc*II, and *Bam*HI.[80] The electrophoretic mobility in 4% polyacrylamide gel of the DNA-mAb $^{125}$I-Br 15-6A complexes released by particular restriction endonucleases was compared with the mobility of the free mAb $^{125}$I-Br 15-6A (Figure 18). The complexes released after digestion with *Eco*RI or *Hinc*II (lanes 1 to 4) were much less mobile than the free form of mAb $^{125}$I-Br 15-6A (lane 6). Digestion of the same amount of chromatin ($10^6$ cells) with *Bam*HI did not release $^{125}$I-Br 15-6A (lane 5). No specific radioactive bands were visualized after digestion with *Bam*HI of chromatin prepared from $2 \times 10^6$ cells (lane 6). Some aggregated, high molecular weight material was observed on the top of lane 6. We cannot eliminate the possibility that some *Bam*HI-large fragments do not enter the gel. The difference in mobility of the mAb $^{125}$I-Br 15-6A-bound chromatin fragments ob-

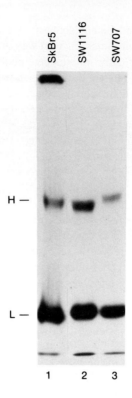

**FIGURE 17.**  Autoradiogram of SDS-polyacrylamide gel electrophoresis (12% polyacrylamide gel) of mAb $^{125}$I-Br 15-6A heavy (H) and light (L) chain incorporated into the chromatin of different tumor cell lines after 24 h incubation. (From Rakowicz-Szulczynska, E., Steplewski, Z., and Koprowski, H., *Am. J. Pathology,* 141, 937, 1992. With permission.)

tained after digestion with *Eco*RI or *Hin*cII suggest that mAb Br 15-6A binds to specific chromatin regions. Since mAb Br 15-6A immunoprecipitated an 88,000 $M_r$ chromatin protein (Figure 16), we suggest that mAb binds to DNA through the mediation of this protein.

## 5.  Effect of Internalized mAb Br 15-6A on RNA and DNA Synthesis

mAb Br 15-6A added to the cell culture media at a broad range of concentration (1 to 4,000 ng/ml) did not affect RNA synthesis by more than 10%. Low effect on RNA synthesis suggests that mAb Br 15-6A may effect expression of unique genes. However, we cannot eliminate a possibility that fluctuation of RNA synthesis of the range of 10% represents non-specific effects of the mouse IgG.

Analysis of the cell growth in the presence of mAb Br 15-6A (Figure 19) indicated that mAb Br 15-6A tested at the concentration range 0.2 to 5 μg/ml progressively inhibited growth of SKBr 5 cells as indicated by 50% lower [$^3$H]thymidine incorporation into DNA and 20% lower cell number, compared to

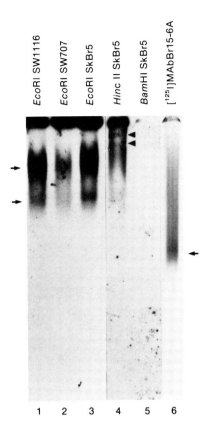

**FIGURE 18.** Electrophoretic analysis and autoradiographic detection (in 4% polyacrylamide gel, nondenaturing conditions) of restriction nuclease-digested chromatin obtained from $10^6$ SKBr5 cells incubated 24 h with mAb $^{125}$I-Br 15-6A. The arrows indicate mAb $^{125}$I-Br 15-6A-bound DNA fragments, which show different electrophoretic mobility than free mAb $^{125}$I-Br 15-6A (lane 6). Digestion with *Bam*HI did not release mAb $^{125}$I-Br 15-6A from the chromatin (lane 5). (From Rakowicz-Szulczynska, E., Steplewski, Z., and Koprowski, H., *Am. J. Pathology*, 141, 937, 1992. With permission.)

the cells not exposed to mAb Br 15-6A. In both colorectal carcinoma cell lines, SW707 and SW1116, mAb Br 15-6A activated growth.

Since the cell surface receptor in SKBr 5 cells exhibits different $M_r$ (92 to 96,000) than in SW707 and SW1116 cells ($M_r$ 108,000) it is likely that opposite effects of this mAb on growth of breast and colorectal carcinoma cell lines are somehow mediated by these two different proteins. We also cannot eliminate the possibility that both lower and higher $M_r$ antigens originate from a single, differently processed or mutated gene.

## D. CONCLUSIONS

The observation that only one of two mAb able to bind to the same cell surface Y antigen is able to penetrate the cell and transport the radioactive ligand to the

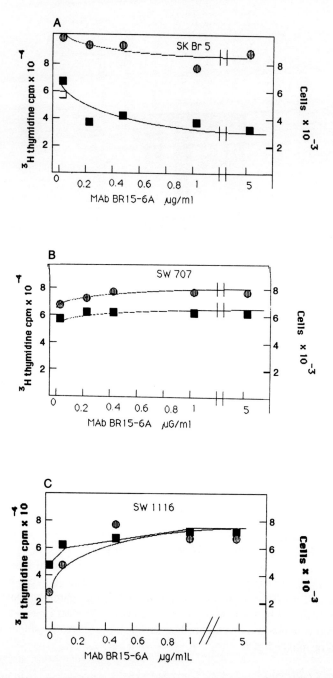

**FIGURE 19.** Effect of mAb Br 15-6A against carbohydrate Y determinant on proliferation of SKBr 5 breast carcinoma and SW707 and SW1116 colorectal carcinoma cells. Cells were exposed for 4 d to different concentrations of mAb Br 15-6A in the absence or presence of [³H]thymidine. Proliferation of cells was measured as radioactivity incorporation into DNA (■) or the cell number (●).

## Internalization of MAbBr15-6A

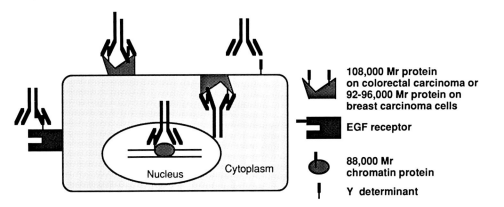

MAb BR 15-6A binds to carbohydrate Y determinant associated with :

- Lipids
- EGF receptor
- 108 kDa cell surface protein (colorectal carcinoma)
- 92-96kDa cell surface protein (breast carcinoma)

**FIGURE 20.** Hypothetical mechanism of mAb Br 15-6A action. mAb Br 15-6A binds to the cell surface carbohydrate Y determinant expressed as glycolipid of glycoprotein. Binding of mAb Br 15-1A to glycolipid does not result in internalization. Recognition of the Y epitope associated with EGF also does not induce internalization. Only binding of mAb Br 15-6A to the 108,000 $M_r$ glycoprotein (in colon carcinoma) or 92,000 to 96,000 $M_r$ glycoprotein in breast carcinoma cells induces internalization. Internalized mAb Br 15-6A is taken up by the nucleus and binds to the nuclear antigen.

chromatin stresses the importance of studies on mAb internalization prior to any clinical usage. Internalization studies may potentially eliminate several cell surface-acting mAb from the radiotherapy, but they do allow identifying the less harmful and most effective mAb for the therapy. For example, knowledge of the mechanisms of mAb Br 15-6A (Figure 20) and mAb Br 55-2 interaction with target cells would allow correct classification of mAb Br 15-6A for the potential radiotherapy (as a carrier of a radioactive ligand) while eliminating mAb Br 55-2 from such a therapy. mAb Br 55-2 is useless as a carrier of a radioactive or a toxin ligand since it binds only to the cell surface, while it represents a good mAb for induction of cell surface reactions, such as antibody-dependent cellular cytotoxicity or antibody-dependent complement-mediated cytolysis.

The fact that the internalized mAb Br 15-6A exerts an opposite effect on the growth of different tumor cell lines (inhibiting growth of breast carcinoma and promoting growth of colorectal carcinoma) strongly indicates that antigens recognized by a single monoclonal antibody may play a completely different function in particular tumors.

Of several mAbs tested in our laboratory, mAb Br 15-6A is the only mAb against the carbohydrate domain, which is internalized. As we discussed above, it is likely that the carbohydrate Y determinant represents only a part of the epitope recognized by this antibody. Hellström et al.[125] developed two mAb against the carbohydrate Le$^y$ determinant which interact and are selectively internalized by carcinomas of the colon, breast, ovary, and lung. The authors[125] also suggest that Le$^y$ determinant must represent a fragment of the epitopes recognized by the internalized antibodies. Since in general mAb against carbohydrate epitopes are poorly internalized, this group of mAb makes poor vehicles for radioactive or toxin ligands.

# III. PERSPECTIVES OF CANCER IMMUNOTHERAPY WITH INTERNALIZABLE ANTIBODIES

## A. INTRACELLULAR PATHWAYS OF INTERNALIZED mAb

Internalization and nuclear translocation of mAb represents an experimentally observed phenomenon that is extremely difficult to explain in the light of our classical and dogmatic knowledge of the mechanisms of protein sorting within the cell. It seems that a very unique conformational interaction of the antibody with the specific epitope of the cell surface antigen induces endocytosis of mAb. The protein antigen, able to mediate internalization of a mAb, behaves like a cell surface receptor which participates in endocytosis of a growth factor. We may suspect that the internalization-mediating antigen represents in fact a receptor for the yet unknown ligand. Such an antigen (receptor) has a natural ability to internalize specific ligands which are likely to represent growth factors or other regulatory proteins. mAb directed against such a cell surface antigen represents an "artificial" ligand which, after binding to the epitope recognized also by the natural ligand, induces internalization of the antigen-ligand complex. Thus, mAb is taken up into the cell instead of the original ligand (growth factor or another regulatory factor). However, in order to be internalized, the antibody has to recognize a very specific domain of the antigen. Binding to a protein domain different than that mediating internalization protects the receptor from internalization, and the antibody remains on the cell surface. Typical examples of the former case are mAb ME 20.4 and mAb ME 82.11, both of which bind to the NGF cell surface receptor (87) at a region different than that recognized by NGF. As a consequence, neither mAb is internalized, although the original ligand (NGF) exhibits an easy entry into the cells. Another receptor for a typical growth factor is the EGF receptor, which mediates internalization of mAb 425 against a protein domain of this receptor, but not of mAb Br15-6A against the carbohydrate domain of this receptor. The fact that the cell surface antigen (receptor) — which, in natural circumstances, binds a low-molecular weight ligand as a growth factor — when bound to a mAb or a mAb-toxin conjugate of a much higher molecular weight induces endocytosis of the whole complex, strongly suggests that activation of a specific domain of the cell surface receptor is more important in induction of internalization than the size of the ligand.

How, after internalization, the antibody is separated from the cell surface receptor inside the cell and how it is released from the cytoplasmic membrane system remains unclear. That the antibody is somehow released from the lysosomes is directly proved by the observation that subunit A of the ricin toxin covalently bound to an antibody is able to penetrate the cytosol and interact with ribosomes. mAb internalized by the cell appears inside the nucleus as a free (of the cell surface antigen) and nondegraded molecule which binds tightly and specifically to the chromatin. How the antibody penetrates the nucleus represents a mystery which also requires further studies. Experimental data suggest that different mAb penetrate the nucleus in different ways: some seem to use the lectin-inhibited nuclear pore complex receptor; others use a specific nuclear membrane-bound antigen or unknown channels; and the rest seem to require activation by the cell surface antigen-binding or an undefined cytoplasmic component prior to the nuclear translocation. mAbs which entered the cytoplasm were also found in the nucleus bound to a specific chromatin antigen, which could be immunoprecipitated by that antibody. Only one mAb against breast carcinoma cells was found to detect the same antigen on the cell surface and in the chromatin. All other internalizable mAb immunoprecipitate two electrophoretically distinguishable proteins from the membrane and from the chromatin. The fact that nuclear translocation and chromatin binding follow internalization of mAb sheds a new light on the role of receptor-ligand endocytosis. Our experiments indicate that internalization through the receptor-mediated endocytosis of the ligand (mAb) does not represent the last step of the ligand's life preceding the lysosomal degradation, but instead represents only a first step in a chain of molecular events that follow ligand entry into the cell. A significant fraction of the internalized mAb in a non-degraded form enters the nucleus and binds to a specific chromatin antigen, while another fraction remains in the cytosol and interacts with the *de novo* synthesized, polysome-bound antigen. The number of antibody molecules that penetrate the nucleus varies for particular antibodies from a few to more than 100,000. The ratio between the number of mAb molecules accumulated in the cytoplasm and the number of molecules taken up by the nucleus is specific for the given mAb and the particular cell line. The last observation suggests that the mechanism of the nuclear translocation is somehow very precisely controlled. We may suspect that inside the cell, the internalized mAb is using a natural pathway of the original ligand (growth factor). Inside the nucleus, mAb seems to occupy the antigen (receptor) recognized by the original ligand.

Chromatin-bound $^{125}$I-mAb are detected within specific restriction fragments of the chromatin. Thus binding of mAb to the chromatin must be precisely controlled, probably by the localization of chromatin antigens. What are the chromatin antigens recognized by antibodies directed against the cell surface antigens? The existence of nuclear antigens which bind mAb translocated to the nucleus cannot be ignored, although none of the genes for those antigens have been cloned. High cytotoxic potency of $^{125}$I-labeled mAb translocated to the nucleus of tumor cells had already been proven.

## B. DRUG DELIVERY TO THE CELL NUCLEUS — mAb AS VEHICLES

Discovery of a nuclear pathway of internalized mAb suggests that a new class of drugs acting on the DNA level may be simply developed. mAb which provide vehicles for this new generation of drugs already exist in several laboratories, but an inappropriate screening using the cell surface binding tests eliminates very often the best candidate mAb from the therapy. In the best cases, immunotoxins are prepared without prior screening for how many mAb molecules, if any, penetrate the cell cytoplasm. Poorly internalized mAb make inefficiently acting immunotoxins. In contrast, internalizable antibodies disappearing from the surface of tumor cells may decrease efficiency of antibody-mediated cellular cytotoxicity or antibody-dependent complement-mediated cytolysis. Finally, uncontrolled growth-stimulating effects of the mAb translocated to the nucleus cannot be predicted without careful evaluation of mAb intracellular interaction. Internalizable mAb may stimulate (or inhibit) expression of the cell surface antigen which in some cases may lead to tumor cell growth activation. Internalization and nuclear translocation represent the biological facts which have to be taken into consideration in drug development, even if our knowledge does not find the answer for the mechanisms of these phenomena.

# REFERENCES

1. **Bast, R. C., Jr., Klug, T. L., St. Johm, E., Jenison, E., Niloff, J. M., Lazarus, M., Berkowitz, R., Leavitt, S., Griffiths, T., Parker, L., Zurawski, V. R., and Knapp, R. C.,** A radioimmunoassay using a monoclonal antibody to monitor the course of epithelial ovarian cancer, *N. Engl. J. Med.,* 309, 883, 1983.

2. **Steplewski, Z., Chans, T. H., Herlyn, M., and Koprowski, H.,** Release of monoclonal antibody-defined antigens by human colorectal carcinoma and melanoma cells, *Cancer Res.,* 41, 2723, 1981.

3. **Higashi, H., Hirabayashi, Y., Hirota, M., Matsumoto, M., and Kato, S.,** Detection of ganglioside GM2 in sera and tumor tissues of hepatoma patients, *Jpn. J. Cancer Res.,* 78, 1309, 1987.

4. **Houghton, A. N., Mintzer, D., Cordon-Cardo, C., Welt, S., Fliegel, B., Vadhen, S., Carswell, E., Melamcol, M. R., Oettgen, M. F., and Ulof, L.,** Mouse monoclonal IgG3 antibody detecting $G_{D3}$ ganglioside: a phase I trial in patients with malignant melanoma, *Proc. Natl. Acad. Sci. U.S.A.,* 82, 1242, 1985.

5. **Koprowski, H., Herlyn, M., and Steplewski, Z.,** Specific antigen in serum of patients with colon carcinoma, *Science,* 212, 53, 1981.

6. **Ross, A. H., Herlyn, M., Ernst, C. S., Guerry, D., Bennicelli, J., Ghrist, B. F. D., Atkinson, B., and Koprowski, H.,** Immunoassay for melanoma-associated proteoglycan in the sera of patients using monoclonal and polyclonal antibodies, *Cancer Res.,* 44, 4642, 1984.

7. **Sears, H. F., Atkinson, B., Mattis, J., and Koprowski, H.,** Phase I clinical trial of monoclonal antibody in treatment of gastrointestinal tumors, *Lancet,* 1, 72, 1982.

8. **Sears, H. F., Herlyn, D., Steplewski, Z., and Koprowski, H.,** Phase II clinical trial of a murine monoclonal antibody cytotoxic for gastrointestinal adenocarcinoma, *Cancer Res.,* 45, 5910, 1985.

9. **Sears, H. F., Herlyn, D., Steplewski, Z., and Koprowski, H.,** Initial trial: use of murine monoclonal antibodies as immunotherapeutic agents for gastrointestinal adenocarcinomas, *Hybridoma,* 5, 109, 1986.

10. **Takahashi, H., Herlyn, D., Atkinson, B., Powe, J., Rodeck, U., Alavi, A., Bruce, D. A., and Koprowski, H.,** Radioimmunodetection of human glioma xenografts by monoclonal antibody to epidermal growth factor receptor, *Cancer Res.,* 47, 3847, 1987.

11. **Wikstrand, C. J., McLendon, R. E., Bullard, D. E., Fredman, P., Suennerholm, L., and Bigner, D. D.**, Production and characterization of two human glioma xenograft-localizing monoclonal antibodies, *Cancer Res.,* 46, 5933, 1986.

12. **Herlyn, D. and Koprowski, H.**, IgG2a monoclonal antibodies inhibit human tumor growth through interaction with effector cells, *Proc. Natl. Acad. Sci. U.S.A.,* 79, 4761, 1982.

13. **Sears, H. F., Herlyn, D., Steplewski, Z., and Koprowski, H.**, Effects of monoclonal antibody immunotherapy on patients with gastro-intestinal adenocarcinoma, *J. Biol. Response Mod.,* 3, 138, 1984.

14. **Bullard, D. E. and Bigner, D. D.**, Application of monoclonal antibodies in the diagnosis and treatment of primary brain tumors, *J. Neurosurg.,* 63, 2, 1985.

15. **Epenetos, A. A., Courtenay-Luck, N., Pickering, D., Hooker, G., Durbin, H., Lavender, J. P., and McKenzie, C. G.**, Antibody guided irradiation of brain glioma by arterial infusion of radioactive monoclonal antibody against epidermal growth factor receptor and blood group A antigen, *Br. Med. J.,* 290, 1463, 1985.

16. **Lee, Y. and Bigner, D. D.**, Aspects of immunobiology and immunotherapy and uses of monoclonal antibodies and biologic immune modifiers in human glioma, *Neurol. Clin.,* 3, 901, 1985.

17. **Brady, L. W., Markoe, A. M., Woo, V. D., Amendola, B. E., Karlsson, U. L., Rackover, M. A., Koprowski, H., Steplewski, Z., and Peyster, R. G.**, Iodine-125-labeled anti-epidermal growth factor receptor-425 in the treatment of glioblastoma multiforme, *Front. Rad. Ther. Oncol.,* 24, 151, 1990.

18. **Brady, L. W., Woo, D. V., Markow, A., Dadparvar, S., Karlsson, U., Rackover, M., Peyster, R., Emrich, J., Miyamoto, C., Steplewski, Z., and Koprowski, H.**, Treatment of malignant gliomas with $^{125}$I-labeled monoclonal antibody against epidermal growth factor receptor, *Antibody Immunoconjugat. Radiopharm.,* 3, 169, 1990.

19. **Kalofonos, H. P., Pawlikowska, T. R., Hemingway, A., Courtenay-Luck, N., Dhokia, B., Snook, D., Sivolapenko, G. B., Hooker, G. R., McKenzie, C. G., Lavender, P. J., Thomas, D. G. T., and Epenetos, A. A.**, Antibody guided diagnosis and therapy of brain gliomas using radiolabeled monoclonal antibodies against epidermal growth factor receptor and placental alkaline phosphatase, *J. Nucl. Med.,* 30, 1636, 1989.

20. **Humm, J. L.**, Dosimetric aspects of radiolabeled antibodies for tumor therapy, *J. Nucl. Med.,* 27, 1490, 1986.

21. **Siccardi, A. G., Buraggi, G. L., Callegaro, L., Colelle, A. C., De Filippi, P. G., Galli, G., Mariani, G., Masi, R., Palumbo, R., Riva, P., Salvatore, R. M., Scassellati, G. A., Scheidhauer, K., Turco, G. L., Zaniol, P., Benini, S., Deleide, G., Gasparini, M., Lastoria, S., Mansi, L., Paganelli, G., Salvischiani, E., Seregni, E., Viale, G., and Natali, P. G.**, Immunoscintigraphy of adenocarcinomas by means of radiolabeled F(ab')₂ fragments of an anticarcinoembryonic antigen monoclonal antibody: a multicenter study, *Cancer Res.,* 49, 3095, 1989.

22. **Zalutsky, M. R., Moseley, R. P., Benjamin, J. C., Colapinto, E. V., Fuller, G. N., Coakham, H. P., and Bigner, D. D.**, Monoclonal antibody and F(ab')₂ fragment delivery to tumor patients with gliomas: comparison of intracarotid and intravenous administration, *Cancer Res.,* 50, 4105, 1990.

23. **Bender, H., Takahashi, H., Adachi, K., Belser, P., Lieng, S., Prewett, M., Schrappe, M., Sutter, A., Rodeck, U., and Herlyn, D.**, Immunotherapy of human glioma xenografts with unlabeled, $^{131}$I-, or $^{125}$I-labeled monoclonal antibody 425 to epidermal growth factor receptor, *Cancer Res.,* 52, 121, 1992.

24. **Miller, R. A., Maloney, D. G., Warnke, R., and Levy, R.**, Treatment of B-cell lymphoma with monoclonal anti-idiotype antibody, *N. Engl. J. Med.,* 306, 517, 1981.

25. **Sindelar, W. F., Maher, M. M., Herlyn, D., Sears, H. F., Steplewski, Z., and Koprowski, H.**, Trial of therapy with monoclonal antibody 17-1A in pancreatic carcinoma: preliminary results, *Hybridoma,* 5 (Suppl. 1), S125, 1986.

26. **Chatal, J.-F., Saccavini, J.-C., Fumoleau, P., Douillar, J. Y., Curtel, C., Kremer, M., Lemevel, B., and Koprowski, H.**, Immunoscintigraphy of colon carcinoma, *J. Nucl. Med.,* 25, 307, 1984.

27. **Hnatowich, D. J., Griffin, T. W., Kosciuczyk, C., Rusckow, S. M., Childs, R. L., Mattis, J. A., Shely, D., and Doherty, P. W.,** Pharmacokinetics of an indium-11-labeled monoclonal antibody in cancer patients, *J. Nucl. Med.,* 26, 849, 1985.

28. **Munz, D. L., Alavi, A., Koprowski, H., and Herlyn, D.,** Improved radioimmunoimaging of tumor xenografts by a mixture of monoclonal antibody F(ab')₂ fragments, *J. Nucl. Med.,* 27, 1739, 1986.

29. **Shen, J.-W., Atkinson, B., Koprowski, H., and Sears, H. F.,** Binding of murine immunoglobulin to human tissues after immunotherapy with anticolorectal carcinoma monoclonal antibody, *Int. J. Cancer,* 33, 465, 1984.

30. **LoBuglio, A. F., Saleh, M. N., Lee, J., Khazaeli, M. B., Carrano, R., Holden, M., and Wheeler, R. H.,** Phase I trial of multiple large doses of murine monoclonal antibody CO17-1A. I. Clinical aspects, *J. Natl. Cancer Inst.,* 80, 932, 1988.

31. **Frödin, J.-E., Harmenberg, U., Biberfeld, P., Christensson, B., Lefvert, A. K., Rieger, A., Shetye, J., Wahren, B., and Mellstedt, M.,** Clinical effects of monoclonal antibodies (mAb 17-1A) in patients with metastatic colorectal carcinomas, *Hybridoma,* 7, 309, 1988.

32. **Shaw, D., Khazadi, M., Sun, L., Ghrayeb, J., Daddona, P. E., McKinney, S., and LoBuglio, A. F.,** Characterization of a mouse/human chimeric monoclonal antibody (17-1A) to a colon cancer tumor-associated antigen, *J. Immunol.,* 138, 4534, 1987.

33. **Herlyn, D., Sears, H. F., Ernst, C. S., Iliopoulos, D., Steplewski, Z., and Koprowski, H.,** Initial clinical evaluation of two murine IgG2a monoclonal antibodies for immunotherapy of gastrointestinal carcinoma, *Am. J. Clin. Oncol.,* 14(5), 371, 1991.

34. **Blottiere, H. M., Douillard, J. Y., Koprowski, H., and Steplewski, Z.,** Immunoglobulin class and immunoglobulin G subclass analysis of human anti-mouse antibody response during monoclonal antibody treatment of cancer patients, *Cancer Res. Suppl.,* 50, 1051S, 1990.

35. **Herlyn, D., Herlyn, M., Steplewski, Z., and Koprowski, H.,** Monoclonal antibodies in cell-mediated cytotoxicity against human melanoma and colorectal carcinoma, *Eur. J. Immunol.,* 9, 657, 1979.

36. **Herlyn, D., Steplewski, Z., Herlyn, M., and Koprowski, H.,** Inhibition of growth of colorectal carcinoma in nude mice by monoclonal antibody, *Cancer Res.,* 40, 717, 1980.

38. **Herlyn, M., Thurin, J., Balaban, G., Bennicelli, J. C., Herlyn, D., Elder, D. E., Bondi, E., Guerry, D., Nowell, P. C., Clark, W. H., and Koprowski, H.,** Characteristics of cultured human melanocytes isolated from different stages of tumor progression, *Cancer Res.,* 45, 5670, 1985.

39. **Herlyn, D., Linnenbach, A., Koprowski, H., and Herlyn, M.,** Epitope- and antigen-specific cancer vaccines, *Int. Rev. Immunol.,* 7, 245, 1991.

40. **Ross, A. H., Herlyn, D., Steplewski, Z., and Koprowski, H.,** Monoclonal antibodies as applied to tumor-associated antigens in the CO17-1A antigen, in *Human Immunogenetics,* Litwin, S. D., Ed., Marcel Dekker, New York, 1987, 107.

41. **Nanda, A., Liwnicz, B., Atkinson, B. F., Sela, B.-A., Takahashi, H., Belser, P. H., Black, P., Koprowski, H., and Herlyn, D.,** Monoclonal antibodies with cytotoxic reactivities against human gliomas, *J. Neurosurg.,* 71, 892, 1989.

42. **Herlyn, D., Sears, H. F., Ernst, C. S., Iliopoulos, D., Steplewski, Z., and Koprowski, H.,** Initial clinical evaluation of two murine IgG2a monoclonal antibodies for immunotherapy of gastrointestinal carcinoma, *Am. J. Clin. Oncol. (CCT),* 14, 371, 1991.

43. **Shawler, D. L., Bartholomew, R. M., Smith, L. M., Dillman, R. O.,** Human immune response to multiple injections of murine monoclonal IgG, *Immunol.,* 135, 1530, 1985.

44. **Olsson, L. and Kaplan, H. S.,** Human-human hybridomas producing monoclonal antibodies of predefined antigenetic specificity, *Proc. Natl. Acad. Sci. U.S.A.,* 77, 5429, 1980.

45. **Larnick, J. W., and Bourla, J. M.,** Prospects for the therapeutic use of human monoclonal antibodies, *J. Biol. Resp. Med.,* 5, 379, 1986.

46. **Morrison, S. L., Johnson, M. J., Herzenberg, L. A., and Oi, V. T.,** Chimeric human antibody molecules make antigen-binding domains with human construct region domains, *Proc. Natl. Acad. Sci. U.S.A.,* 81, 6851, 1984.

47. **Sahagan, B., Dorai, H., Saltzgaber-Muller, J., Toneguzzo, F., Guindon, C., Lilly, S., McDonald, K., Morrissey, D., Stone, B., Davis, G., McIntosh, P., and Moore, G. P.,** A genetically engineered murine/human chimeric antibody retains specificity for human tumor-associated antigen, *J. Immunol.,* 137, 1066, 1986.

48. **Nishimure, Y., Yokoyama, M., Aveli, K., Vedo, R., Kurdo, A., and Watanabe, T.,** Recombinant human-mouse chimeric monoclonal antibody specific for common acute lymphocytic leukemic antigen, *Cancer Res.,* 47, 999, 1987.

49. **Sun, L. U., Curtis, P., Rakowicz-Szulczynska, E., Ghrayeb, J., Cheng, N., Morrison, S. L., and Koprowski, H.,** Chimeric antibody with human constant regions and mouse variable regions directed against carcinoma-associated antigen 17-1A, *Proc. Natl. Acad. Sci. U.S.A.,* 84, 214, 1987.

50. **Koprowski, H., Herlyn, D., Lubeck, M., DeFreitas, E., and Sears, H. F.,** Human anti-idiotype antibodies in cancer patients: is the modulation of the immune response beneficial for the patient?, *Proc. Natl. Acad. Sci. U.S.A.,* 81, 216, 1984.

51. **Herlyn, D., Ross, A. H., and Koprowski, H.,** Anti-idiotypic antibodies bear the internal image of a human tumor antigen, *Science,* 232, 100, 1986.

52. **Koprowski, H.,** Significance of anti-idiotype antibodies in cancer patients, in *Monographs in Allergy,* Dukor, P., Manson, L. A., Kallos, P., Shakib, F., Tinka, Z., Walesman, B. A., Eds., Vol. 22, S. Karger, Basel, 1987, 180.

53. **Vitetta, E. S., and Krolick, K. A., Miyama-Inaba, M., Cushley, W., and Uhr, J. W.,** Immunotoxins: a new approach to cancer therapy, *Science,* 219, 644, 1983.

54. **Blakey, D. C. and Thorpe, P. E.,** An overview of therapy with immunotoxins containing ricin or its A chain, *Antibody Immunoconj. Radiopharm.,* 1, 1, 1988.

55. **Ross, W. C., Thorpe, P. E., Cumber, A. J., Edwards, D. C., Hinson, C. A., and Davis, A. J.,** Increased toxicity of diphtheria toxin for human lymphoblastoid cells following covalent linkage for anti-(human lymphocyte) globulin or its F(ab')$_2$ fragment, *Eur. J. Biochem.,* 104, 381, 1980.

56. **Endo, Y., Mitsui, K., Matizuki, M., and Tsurugi, K.,** The mechanisms of action of ricin and related toxic lectins on eukaryotic ribosomes, *J. Biol. Chem.,* 202, 5908, 1987.

57. **Endo, Y. and Tsurugi, K.,** RNA N-glycosidase activity of ricin A chain. Mechanism of action of the toxic lectin ricin on eukaryotic ribosomes, *J. Biol. Chem.,* 262, 8128, 1987.

58. **Gilliland, D. G., Steplewski, Z., Collier, R. Y., Mitchell, K. F., Chang, T. M., and Koprowski, H.,** Antibody-directed cytotoxic agents: use of monoclonal antibody to direct the action of toxin A chains to colorectal carcinoma cells. *Proc. Natl. Acad. Sci. U.S.A.,* 77, 4539, 1980.

59. **Spitler, L. E., del Rio, M., Khentigan, A., Wedel, N. L., Brophy, N. A., Miller, L. L., Harkonen, W. S., Rosendorf, L. L., Lee, H. M., Mischak, R. P., Kawahata, R. T., Stoudemire, J. B., Fradkin, L. B., Bautista, E. E., and Scannon, P. J.,** Therapy of patients with malignant melanoma using a monoclonal antimelanoma antibody-ricin A chain immunotoxin, *Cancer Res.,* 47, 1717, 1987.

60. **Embleton, M. J., Byers, V. S., Lee, H. M., Scannon, P. J., Blackhall, N. W., and Baldwin, R. W.,** Sensitivity and selectivity of ricin toxin A chain monoclonal antibody 791T/36 conjugates against human tumor cell lines, *Cancer Res.,* 46, 5524, 1986.

61. **Bjorn, M. J., Ring, D., and Frankel, A.,** Evaluation of monoclonal antibodies for the development of breast cancer immunotoxins, *Cancer Res.,* 45, 1214, 1985.

62. **Pirker, R., Fitzgerald, J. P., Hamilton, R. C., Ozols, R. F., Laird, W., Frankel, A. E., Willingham, M. C., and Pastan, I.,** Characterization of immunotoxins active against ovarian cancer cell lines, *J. Clin. Invest.,* 76, 1261, 1985.

63. **Canevari, S., Orlandi, R., Ripamonti, M., Tagliabue, E., Aguanno, S., Miott, S., Menard, S., and Colnaghi, M. I.,** Ricin A chain conjugated with monoclonal antibodies selectively killing human carcinoma cells *in vitro, J. Natl. Cancer Inst.,* 75, 831, 1985.

64. **Griffin, T. W., Richardson, C., Houston, L. L., LePage, D., Bogden, A., and Raso, V.,** Antitumor activity of intraperitoneal immunotoxins in a nude mouse model of human malignant mesothelioma, *Cancer Res.,* 47, 4266, 1987.

65. **Byers, V. S., Rodvien, R., Grant, K., Durrant, L. G., Hudson, K. H., Baldwin, R. W., and Scannon, P. J.,** Phase I study of monoclonal antibody-ricin A chain immunotoxin XomaZyme-791 in patients with metastatic colon cancer, *Cancer Res.,* 49, 6153, 1989.

66. **Jansen, F. K., Blythman, H. E., Carriere, D., Cosellas, P., Gros, D., Gros, P., Langent, J. C., Pastucci, F., Pan, B., Poucelet, P., Richer, G., Videl, M., and Voisin, G. A.,** Immunotoxins — hybrid molecules combining high specificity and potent cyto-toxicity, *Immunol. Rev.,* 62, 185, 1982.

67. **Houston, L. L. and Norinski, R. C.,** Cell-specific cytotoxicity expressed by a conjugate of ricin and murine monoclonal antibody directed against Thy 1.1 antigen, *Cancer Res.,* 41, 3913, 1981.

68. **Oeltmann, T. N. and Forbes, J. T.,** Inhibition of mouse spleen cell function by dipheric toxin fragment A coupled to anti-mouse Thy 1.2 and by ricin A chain coupled to anti-mouse IgM, *Arch. Biochem. Biophys.,* 209, 362, 1981.

69. **Kernan, N. A., Knowles, R. W., Burns, M. J., Broxmeyer, H. E., Lu, L., Lee, H. M., Kawahata, R. T., Scannon, P. J., and Dupont, B.,** Specific inhibition of *in vitro* lymphocyte transformation by an anti-pan T cell (gp6) ricin A chain immunotoxin, *J. Immunol.,* 133, 137, 1984.

70. **Martin, P. J., Hansen, J. A., and Vitetta, E. S.,** A ricin A chain-containing immunotoxin that kills human T lymphocytes *in vitro, Blood,* 66, 908, 1985.

71. **Laurent, G., Paris, J., Farcet, J. P., Carayon, P., Blythman, H., Casellas, F., Poncelet, P., and Jansen, F. K.,** Effects of therapy with T101-ricin A chain immunotoxin in two leukemia patients, *Blood,* 67, 1680, 1986.

72. **Katz, F. E., Janossy, G., Cumber, A., Ross, W., Blacklock, H. A., Tax, W., and Thorpe, P. E.,** Elimination of T cells from human peripheral blood and bone marrow using a cocktail of three anti-T cell immunotoxins, *Br. J. Haematol.,* 67, 407, 1987.

73. **Kargen, B. L., Finkelstein, A., and Colombini, M.,** Diphtheria toxin fragment forms large pores in phospholipid bilayer membranes, *Proc. Natl. Acad. Sci. U.S.A.,* 78, 4950, 1981.

74. **Byers, V. S., Henslee, P. J., Kernan, N. A., Blazar, B. R., Gingrich, R., Phillips, G. L., LeMaistre, C. F., Gilliland, G., Antin, J. H., Martin, P., Tutscha, P. J., Trown, P. W., Ackerman, S. K., O'Reilly, R. J., and Scannon, P. J.,** Use of anti-pan T-lymphocyte ricin A chain immunotoxin in steroid-resistant acute graft-versus-host disease, *Blood,* 75, 1426, 1990.

75. **Kernan, N. A., Byers, V. S., Scannon, P. J., Mishak, R. P., Brochstein, J., Flomenberg, N., Dupont, B., and O'Reilly, R. J.,** Treatment of steroid-resistant acute graft-versus-host disease by *in vivo* administration of anti-T cell ricin A chain immunotoxin, *J. Am. Med. Assoc.,* 259, 3154, 1987.

76. **Blakey, D. C., Wawrzynczak, E. J., Wallace, P. M., and Thorpe, P. E.,** Antibody toxin conjugates: a perspective, *Prog. Allergy,* 45, 50, 1988.

77. **Trown, P. W., Reardan, D. T., Carroll, S. F., Stoudemire, J. B., and Kawahata, R. T.,** Improved pharmacokinetics and tumor localization of immunotoxins constructed with the $M_r$ 30,000 form of ricin A chain, *Cancer Res.,* 51, 4219, 1991.

78. **Rakowicz-Szulczynska, E., Otwiaski, D., Rodeck, U., and Koprowski, H.,** Epidermal growth factor (EGF) and monoclonal antibody to cell surface EGF receptor bind to the same chromatin receptor, *Arch. Biochem. Biophys.,* 268, 456, 1989.

79. **Rakowicz-Szulczynska, E. and Koprowski, H.,** Nuclear uptake of monoclonal antibody to a surface glycoprotein and its effect on transcription, *Arch. Biochem. Biophys.,* 271, 366, 1989.

80. **Rakowicz-Szulczynska, E., Steplewski, Z., and Koprowski, H.,** Nuclear translocation of monoclonal antibody directed against cell surface carbohydrate Y determinant, *Am. J. Pathology,* 141, 937, 1992.

81. **Rakowicz-Szulczynska, E. and Koprowski, H.,** U.S. patent application.

82. **Rakowicz-Szulczynska, E., Rodeck, U., Herlyn, M., and Koprowski, H.,** Chromatin binding of epidermal growth factor, nerve growth factor, and platelet-derived growth factor in cells bearing the appropriate surface receptors, *Proc. Natl. Acad. Sci. U.S.A.,* 83, 3728, 1986.

83. **Rakowicz-Szulczynska, E. and Koprowski, H.**, Identification of NGF receptor in chromatin of melanoma cells using monoclonal antibody to cell surface NGF receptor, *Biochem. Biophys. Res. Commun.*, 140, 174, 1986.
84. **Rakowicz-Szulczynska, E.**, Identification of the cell surface and nuclear receptors for NGF in a breast carcinoma cell line, *J. Cell Physiol.*, 154, 71, 1993.
85. **Rakowicz-Szulczynska, E., Herlyn, M., and Koprowski, H.**, Nerve growth factor receptors in chromatin of melanoma cells, proliferating melanocytes, and colorectal carcinoma cells *in vitro, Cancer Res.*, 48, 7200, 1988.
86. **Rakowicz-Szulczynska, E., Reddy, V., Vorbrodt, A., Herlyn, D., and Koprowski, H.**, Chromatin and cell surface receptor mediate melanoma cell growth response to nerve growth factor, *Mol. Carcinogenesis*, 4, 388, 1991.
87. **Ross, A. H., Grob, P., Bothwell, M., Elder, D. E., Ernst, C. S., Marano, M., Ghrist, B. F. D., Slemp, C. C., Herlyn, M., Atkinson, B., and Koprowski, H.**, Characterization of nerve growth factor receptor in neural crest tumors using monoclonal antibodies, *Proc. Natl. Acad. Sci. U.S.A.*, 81, 6681, 1984.
88. **Murthy, V., Basu, A., Rodeck, U., Herlyn, M., Ross, A., and Das, M.**, Domain-specificity and antagonistic properties of a new monoclonal antibody to the EGF-receptor, *Arch. Biochem. Biophys.*, 252, 549, 1987.
89. **Atkinson, B., Ernst, C. S., Ghrist, B. F. D., Herlyn, M., Blaszczyk, M., Ross, A. H., Herlyn, D., Steplewski, Z., and Koprowski, H.**, Identification of melanoma-associated antigens using fixed tissue screening of antibodies, *Cancer Res.*, 44, 2577, 1984.
90. **Hotta, H., Ross, A. H., Huebner, K., Isobe, M., Wendeborn, S., Chao, M. V., Ricciardi, R. P., Tsujimoto, Y., Croce, C., and Koprowski, H.**, Molecular cloning and characterization of an antigen associated with early stages of melanoma tumor progression, *Cancer Res.*, 48, 2955, 1988.
91. **Herlyn, M.**, unpublished data.
92. **Wistar Institute**, unpublished data.
93. **Rakowicz-Szulczynska, E.**, manuscript in preparation.
94. **Herlyn, M., Steplewski, Z., Herlyn, D., and Koprowski, H.**, Colorectal carcinoma-specific antigen: detection by means of monoclonal antibodies, *Proc. Nat. Acad. Sci. U.S.A.*, 76, 1938–1979.
95. **Ross, A. M., Herlyn, D., Iliopoulos, D., and Koprowski, H.**, Isolation and characterization of a carcinoma-associated antigen, *Biochem. Biophys. Res. Commun.*, 135, 297, 1986.
96. **Woo, D., Li, D., Mattis, J., and Steplewski, Z.**, Selective chromosomal damage and cytotoxicity of $^{125}I$-labeled monoclonal antibody 17-1A in human cancer cells, *Cancer Res.*, 49, 2952, 1989.
97. **Herlyn, M., Steplewski, Z., Herlyn, D., and Koprowski, H.**, Related monoclonal antibodies — their production and characterization, *Hybridoma*, 5, 51, 1986.
98. **Linnenbach, A. J., Wojcierowski, J., Wu, S., Pyrc, J. J., Ross, A. H., Dietzschold, B., Speicher, D., and Koprowski, H.**, Sequence investigation of the major gastrointestinal tumor-associated antigen gene family, GA 733, *Proc. Natl. Acad. Sci. U.S.A.*, 86, 27, 1989.
99. **Thurin, M., Thurin, J., Hindsgaul, O., Karlsson, K. A., Steplewski, Z., and Koprowski, H.**, Y and blood group B type glycolipid antigens accumulate in human gastric carcinoma cell line as detected by monoclonal antibody, *J. Biol. Chem.*, 262, 372, 1987.
100. **Basu, M., Murthy, U., Rodeck, U., Herlyn, M., Mattis, L., and Das, M.**, Presence of tumor-associated antigens in epidermal growth factor receptors from different human carcinomas, *Cancer Res.*, 47, 2531, 1987.
101. **Koprowski, H., Steplewski, Z., Mitchell, V., Herlyn, M., Herlyn, D., and Fuhrer, P.**, Colorectal carcinoma antigens detected by hybridoma antibodies, *Somat. Cell. Genet.*, 5, 957, 1979.
102. **Blaszczyk, M., Pak, K. Y., Herlyn, M., Lindgren, Y., Pesseno, S., Steplewski, Z., and Koprowski, H.**, Characterization of gastrointestinal tumor-associated carcinoembryonic antigen-related antigens defined by monoclonal antibodies, *Cancer Res.*, 44, 245, 1984.

103. **Herlyn, M., Blaszczyk, M., Bennicelli, J., Sears, H. F., Ernst, C. S., Ross, A. H., and Koprowski, H.,** Selection of monoclonal antibodies detecting serodiagnostic human tumor markers, *J. Immunol. Methods.,* 80, 107, 1985.

104. **Brockhaus, M., Magnani, J. Z., Blaszczyk, K. M., Steplewski, Z., Koprowski, H., Karlsson, K. A., Larson, Y., and Ginsburg, V.,** Monoclonal antibodies directed against the human Le$^b$ blood group antigen, *J. Biol. Chem.,* 256, 13223, 1981.

105. **Blaszczyk, M., Hansson, O. C., Karlsson, K. A., Larson, G., Strömberg, N., Thurin, J., Herlyn, M., Steplewski, Z., and Koprowski, H.,** Lewis blood group antigens defined by monoclonal anti-colon carcinoma antibodies, *Arch. Biochem. Biophys.,* 233, 161, 1984.

106. **Thurin, J.,** unpublished data.

107. **Steplewski, Z.,** unpublished data.

108. **Steplewski, Z.,** unpublished data.

109. **Rakowicz-Szulczynska, E., Linnenbach, A. J., and Koprowski, H.,** Intracellular receptors binding and nuclear transport of NGF in intact cells and a cell-free system, *Mol. Carcinogenesis,* 2, 47, 1989.

110. **Rakowicz-Szulczynska, E. and Koprowski, H.,** Antagonistic effect of NGF and PDGF on ribosomal RNA systems and tumor cell proliferation, *Biochem. Biophys. Res. Commun.,* 163, 649, 1989.

111. **Park, M. K., D'Onofrio, M., Willingham, M. C., and Hanover, J. A.,** A monoclonal antibody against a family of nuclear pore proteins (nucleoporins): O-linked N-acetylglucosamine is part of the immunodominant, *Proc. Natl. Acad. Sci. U.S.A.,* 84, 6462, 1987.

112. **Markland, W., Smith, A. E., and Roberts, B. L.,** Signal-dependent translocation of Simian virus 40 large T antigen into rat liver nuclei in a cell-free system, *Mol. Cell. Biol.,* 7, 4255, 1987.

113. **Rakowicz-Szulczynska, E., Linnenbach, A., and Koprowski, H.,** Rapid and sensitive method to detect expression of growth factor receptors, *J. Immunol. Methods,* 116, 167, 1989.

114. **Szala, S., Kasai, Y., Steplewski, Z., Rodeck, U., Koprowski, H., and Linnenbach, A. J.,** Molecular cloning of cDNA for the human tumor-associated antigen CO-029 and identification of related transmembrane antigens, *Proc. Natl. Acad. Sci. U.S.A.,* 87, 6833, 1990.

115. **Classon, B. J., Williams, A. F., Willis, A. C., Seed, B., and Stamenkovic, I.,** The primary structure of the human leukocyte antigen CD37, a species homologue of the rat MRC OX-44 antigen, *J. Exp. Med.,* 169, 1497, 1989.

116. **Boucheix, C., Benott, P., Frachet, P., Billard, M., Worthington, R. E., Gagnon, J., and Vzan, G.,** Molecular cloning of the CD9 antigen. A new family of cell surface proteins, *J. Biol. Chem.,* 266, 117, 1991.

117. **Angelisova, P., Vicek, C., Stefanova, I., Lipoldof, M., and Horejsi, V.,** The human leukocyte surface antigen CD53 is a protein structurally similar to the CD37 and MRC OX-44 antigens, *Immunogenetics,* 32, 281, 1990.

118. **Oren, R., Takahashi, S., Doss, C., Levy, R., and Levy, S.,** TAPA-1, the target of an antiproliferative antibody, defines a new family of transmembrane proteins, *Mol. Cell Biol.,* 10, 4007, 1990.

119. **Wright, M. D., Mendele, K. J., and Mitchell, G. F.,** An immunogenic $M_r$ 23,000 integral membrane protein of *Schistosoma mansoni* worms that closely resembles a human tumor-associated antigen, *J. Immunol.,* 144, 195, 1990.

120. **Demetrick, D. J., Herlyn, D., Tretiak, M., Creasey, D., Clevers, H., Donoso, L. A., Vennegoor, C. J. G. M., Dixon, W. T., Jerry, L. M.,** ME 491 melanoma-associated glycoprotein family: antigenic identity of ME 491, NKI/C-3, neuroglandular antigen(NGA), and CD63 proteins, *J. Natl. Cancer Inst.,* 84, 422, 1992.

121. **Bouche, G., Gas, N., Prats, H., Baldin, U., Tauber, J. P., Terssie, J., and Amalvic, F.,** Basic fibroblast growth factor enters the nucleolus and stimulates the transcription of ribosomal genes in ABAE cells undergoing $G_0 \rightarrow G_1$ transition, *Proc. Natl. Acad. Sci. U.S.A.,* 84, 7660, 1982.

122. **Thurin, J.**, Binding sites of monoclonal anti-carbohydrate antibodies, in *Current Topics in Microbiology and Immunology*, Springer-Verlag, Berlin, Heidelberg, 139, 1988, 59–79.

123. **Chen, M. T. and Kabat, E. A.**, Immunological studies of blood groups. The combining site specificities of mouse monoclonal hybridoma anti-A and anti-B, *J. Biol. Chem.*, 260, 13208, 1985.

124. **Lemieux, R. V.**, How oligosacharides are recognized for specific noncovalent binding by antibodies and lectins, in *Proceedings of the VIIIth International Symposium on Glycoconjugates*, Praegen, NY, 177.

125. **Hellström, J., Garrigues, H. J., Garrigues, U., and Hellström, K. E.**, Highly tumor-reactive, internalizing mouse monoclonal antibodies to Le$^y$-related cell surface antigens, *Cancer Res.*, 50, 2183, 1990.

Chapter 5

# INTERNALIZED ANTIBODIES AS A POTENTIAL TOOL AGAINST RETROVIRAL DISEASES

**Ewa M. Rakowicz-Szulczynska, Wojciech Kaczmarski, Kathelyn S. Steimer, Vic Raso, and Paul J. Durda**

## TABLE OF CONTENTS

# I. NEUTRALIZING ANTIBODIES IN HIV-INFECTIONS

The human immunodeficiency virus type 1 (HIV-1) is the etiological agent which causes the acquired immunodeficiency syndrome (AIDS).[1,4] The virus encodes two envelope glycoproteins, gp120 and gp41, which are cleavage products of a precursor gp160 molecule. Proteins gp120 and gp41 are organized in a lipid bilayer. This envelope covers the gag-derived p17 matrix protein and the cone-shaped core hiding the viral ribonucleoprotein.[5,6] The mechanism of HIV-infection follows the pattern of retroviral infection and involves binding of the virus to the target cell surface receptor, injection of the genetic material into the cell, reverse transcription of the viral RNA, penetration of the nucleus, and integration of the viral double-stranded DNA with the human genome. After transcription of the viral RNA and synthesis of the viral proteins, the new viral molecules are formed. The envelope protein gp120 of HIV recognizes the CD4 receptor on lymphocytes, monocytes, and other cells and, therefore, plays a critical role in the process of infection through the receptor-mediated endocytosis, via clathrin-coated pits and vesicles.[7-13] Another mechanism of HIV entry into the cell involves direct fusion of the viral envelope with the cell membrane, which is the process mediated by gp41.[7,13-15] During infection, the core disintegrates and releases the viral ribonucleoprotein through the opening at the fusion site into the cytoplasm. After infection, the viral genome integrates with the host DNA.[16] A consequence of viral envelope protein (gp120) expression on the surface of the infected cell is that noninfected CD4 receptor-positive T lymphocytes are attracted and syncytia are formed.[17]

Neutralizing antibodies produced in a natural human infection are mainly directed against the third hypervariable domain of gp120 of the virus envelope.[18-22] The epitope of the V3 loop seems to be linear and contains[22] amino acids bound by cysteine residues.[20] Synthetic peptides consisting of sequences within this region or fragments of gp120 induce isolate-restricted neutralizing antibody.[23-25] Neutralizing antibodies appearing early in HIV infection are isolate-specific and directed towards the same region of gp120.[18-22] However, with time, the isolate specificity of the response broadens.[26,27]

The mechanism of the response broadening is unclear, but it is speculated that neutralizing antibodies are directed against conformational epitopes of gp120.[26,27] Recently, broadly neutralizing antibodies were obtained which recognize a conserved region (GlyProGlyArgAlaPhe) of the hypervariable neutralizing domain of HIV-1.[28,29] It is suggested that lack of antibodies against this conserved region may result in the poor organism response to HIV-1 infection.

No correlation has yet been demonstrated between neutralizing antibody titers and progression to disease. Several mechanisms of neutralization are considered: (1) blocking virus binding to the receptor, (2) blocking gp41 conformational change and exposure, (3) blocking fusion/endocytosis, (4) blocking uncoating, and (5) affecting a post-uncoating step/affecting transcription.

Some antibodies neutralize the virus without blocking HIV entry to the cells, while others block CD4/gp120 binding but do not neutralize viral infectivity. It is also observed that neutralizing antibodies in some circumstances may enhance infection. The considered mechanism involves Fc receptor-mediated endocytosis of the virus.

In general, controversial findings have been published on the role of neutralizing antibodies, and there is no general answer for how such antibodies neutralize virus.

## II. ANTIBODY ENTRY INTO HIV-INFECTED CELLS

Several laboratories have developed immunotoxins which consist of a monoclonal antibody against CD4 receptors of T lymphocytes or against HIV envelope proteins, gp120 or gp41, and the ricin A subunit.[30-35] Ricin A represents the active component of ricin toxin, which inhibits protein synthesis due to inactivation of the 60 S ribosomal subunit.[36,37] Subunit A does not penetrate the cell in the absence of the ricin B subunit or specific internalized carrier. Internalized mAb conjugated with ricin A- or diphtheric A-subunits of these toxins are used as immunotoxins in experimental cancer therapy[38,39] (also see Chapter 4). mAb against gp120 and gp41, when conjugated with the ricin A subunit, were also found to exert cytotoxic effects on HIV-infected cells,[33-35] which suggests that gp120 (or gp41) expressed on the surface of HIV-infected cells mediates internalization of mAb. An ideal immunotoxin should penetrate the cell easily; therefore, determining the epitopes of gp120 (or gp41) involved in internalization is critical for developing effective immunoconjugates. Based on our experiments with internalizable anti-cancer mAb[40-42] (also see Chapter 4), we suggest that cell-penetrating antibodies also may have some role in virus neutralization. Studies on internalization and intracellular localization of mAb directed against cancer antigens indicates that most of the mAb are translocated to the cell nucleus and bind to the chromatin antigen(s), which exhibits epitopic homology with the cell surface antigen. Following the pattern of experiments on cancer cells[40-42] (see also Chapter 4), we have analyzed the fate of mAb internalized by HIV-1 infected cells and found that nuclear accumulation of those mAb also follows internalization.[43]

### A. INTERNALIZATION OF mAb AGAINST gp120 BY HIV-1-INFECTED T LYMPHOCYTES

Four [125]I-mAb against the overlapping regions of the variable loop of gp120 were incubated with noninfected or HIV-1-infected T lymphocytes (Table 1).[43] mAb 5023 and mAb 5025 (against HIV-1-III$_B$ gp120 amino acid region 308 to 322)[24,25] are from the DuPont Company; mAb 0.5β against the region 308 to 332[44] was kindly provided by Dr. S. Matsushita from the Kumamoto University Medical School in Japan, and MV77 (307 to 328) was kindly supplied by Dr. F. Veronese from Bionetics Research, Inc. None of the mAb were internalized by noninfected T lymphocytes (Table 1).[43] One day after infection, when the syncytia were undetectable, very low internalization of [125]I-mAb 5023 and [125]I-mAb 5025 was detected.[43] Three days after infection, when 50 to 75% of cells formed syncytia, internalization of mAb 5023 was very high (up to 67,000 molecules per cell) (Table

## TABLE 1
## Internalization of $^{125}$I-mAb Against gp120
## after 24-h Incubation with Noninfected
## or HIV-1-Infected T Lymphocytes

| Day after infection[c] | | Molecules per cell[a] SupT1[b] | |
|---|---|---|---|
| | | Cytoplasm | Nucleus |
| Noninfected | 5023 (308–322)[d] | 68 | 78 |
| | 5025 (308–322) | 92 | 61 |
| | VM77 (307–328) | 54 | 23 |
| | 0.5β (308–332) | 22 | 7 |
| 1 | 5023 | 515 ± 50 | 430 ± 45 |
| | 5025 | 153 ± 25 | 560 ± 50 |
| | VM77 | 70 | 60 |
| | 96-16 | 40 | 20 |
| | 0.5β | 30 | 5 |
| 3 | 5023 | 57,000 ± 10,000 | 10,000 ± 2,000 |
| | 5025 | 4,400 ± 1,000 | 2,100 ± 500 |
| | VM77 | 90 | 50 |
| | 0.5β | 35 | 10 |

[a]   Mean + SD from three experiments.
[b]   T lymphocytes-SupT1 infected with HIV-1 (HXB-2).
[c]   Day after infection is the day when the $^{125}$I-mAb was added to the medium.
[d]   Amino acid residues of gp120 recognized by the mAb.

1). mAb 5025, which was developed against the same synthetic peptide as mAb 5023 (amino acids 308 to 322), was internalized in much lower quantities (6500 molecules per cell) than mAb 5023. mAb 0.5β against amino acid region 308 to 332 and VM77 against the 307 to 328 were not internalized (Table 1). Since all four mAb recognize overlapping regions of gp120 — only one mAb (5023) is internalized in large quantities, one mAb (5025) in low quantities, and none of the others is internalized — a passive uptake of mAb 5023 during endocytosis of the virus is unlikely. The possibility of mAb 5023 uptake during HIV-1 integration with T lymphocytes is further eliminated by the fact that during the first day of infection, when the virus is extensively integrated with the cell, mAb 5023 was not internalized. The fact that all mAb are bound to the gp120 expressed on the cell surface of HIV-infected T lymphocytes eliminates a possibility of an adsorption of the cell-membrane-bound antibody to the intracellular organelles during fractionation. Nonspecific internalization of mAb 5023 or mAb 5025 during syncytia formation is also unlikely, since mAb 0.5β and VM77 were not internalized.[43]

Although both mAb 5023 and mAb 5025 were developed against the same synthetic peptides,[24,25] mAb 5023 was internalized much more efficiently than mAb 5025. It is noteworthy that mAb 5023 exhibits high affinity and high neutralizing activity, while mAb 5025 exhibits very low affinity and low neutralizing activity.[25] Both mAb 5023 and mAb 5025 were raised against peptide RIQRGPGRAFVTIGK which corresponds to gp120 amino acid residues 308 to 322. The underlined tripeptide RAF represents the core epitope recognized by both mAb.[25] However, reactivity of mAb 5023 with tetrapeptide GRAF is threefold that with RAF, which suggests that G residue (marked by filled arrowheads) contributes to binding of mAb 5023. mAb 5025 does not react with the G residue. The affinity of mAb 5023 exceeds by several times the affinity of mAb 5025 which suggests that the neutralizing activity correlates with its affinity.[25]

Internalization of mAb 5023 and, to a lesser degree, of mAb 5025 was observed only during the time when syncytia were formed (i.e., 3 d after infection), which suggests that expression of gp120 on the surface of infected cells (which determines interaction of gp120 with CD4) was critical for internalization. When infection of T lymphocytes was done with lower concentrations of inoculum, syncytia were formed after 4, 5, or 6 d (data not shown). Always, internalization of mAb 5023 (and in lesser amounts mAb 5025) paralleled syncytia formation, which confirms the role of gp120 expressed on the cell surface of the infected cells in mediation of internalization. Fractionation of HIV-1 infected cells (3 d of exposure) after incubation with $^{125}$I-mAb 5023 indicated that mAb localized to the cytoplasm and the nucleus. Approximately 57,000 molecules of $^{125}$I-mAb 5023 were localized in the cytoplasm and 10,000 in the chromatin of one cell. In much smaller quantities, $^{125}$I-mAb 5023 also localized to the nucleus. mAb 5023 and mAb 5025 after translocation to the nucleus were tightly attached to the chromatin (these were not extracted with 2M NaCl).

## B. CYTOTOXICITY OF mAb 5023-RICIN A CONJUGATE

mAb 5023 was conjugated with ricin A chain, and this conjugate was incubated with 8E5 cells, a defective HIV-1-infected cell line (Table 2).[43] Protein synthesis measured as [$^3$H]-leucine incorporation was inhibited by 60% by the mAb 5023-ricin A chain conjugate. The effect of the mAb 5023-ricin A on protein synthesis was completely abolished by the addition of an excess of unconjugated mAb 5023. In control experiments, HIV-1-infected cells were treated with a mAb anti-transferrin receptor (anti-TfR) conjugated to ricin A. Anti-TfR-ricin A conjugate inhibited protein synthesis by 96%, and the effect was not abolished by an excess of mAb 5023 (Table 2).

Protein synthesis in control HIV-negative A3.01 cells was affected by anti-TfR-ricin A conjugate, but not by mAb 5023-ricin A conjugate. The results indicate that mAb 5023-ricin A conjugate is specifically internalized by HIV-1 infected cells and inhibits protein synthesis (cytotoxic effect).[44]

Matsushita et al.[34] found that mAb 0.5β, which in our manuscript is described as noninternalizing mAb (Table 1), after conjugation with ricin A subunit also efficiently kills HIV-infected cells. Since a single molecule of ricin A is sufficient to block protein synthesis, theoretically, an internalization of single molecules (in our experiments, 45 molecules of mAb 0.5β/cell) of the vehicle-mAb is sufficient

## TABLE 2
## Cytotoxicity of mAb 5023-Ricin A Conjugate

|  | [³H]-leucine incorporation (cpm) | Inhibition (%) |
|---|---|---|
| **HIV + 8E5 cells plus** |  |  |
| No additions | 41,785 | 0 |
| mAb 5023-ricin A | 16,850 | 60 |
| mAb 5023-ricin A + excess anti-HIV (5023) | 43,295 | 0 |
| Anti-TfR-A | 1,705 | 96 |
| Anti-TfR-A + excess-anti-HIV | 2,190 | 95 |
| **HIV + A3.01 cells plus** |  |  |
| No additions | 55,770 | 0 |
| mAb 5023-ricin A | 55,430 | 1 |
| Anti-TfR-A | 9,860 | 82 |

to deliver the toxin into the cells. mAb 5023, which is extensively internalized (67,000 molecules/cell), might potentially be used for a very effective delivery of toxins or other more specific drugs into HIV-infected cells. Since we detected 67,000 molecules of $^{125}$I-mAb 5023 per cell, and no more than 45 of mAb 0.5b, mAb 5023-ricin A conjugates could be used in a very low concentration (theoretically 1000-fold lower than that of 0.5b), which would decrease a strong immune reaction toward the ricin A. Harrison et al.[45] constructed a DNA plasmid that expresses a diphtheria toxin A chain gene under control of HIV-1 proteins Tat and Rev. The method presented by Harrison et al.[45] represents one of many novel approaches to AIDS therapy, using "intracellular immunization".[46] Our observations that the HIV-1 envelope protein gp120, when expressed on the target cell, may very effectively mediate internalization of a specific mAb sheds additional light on the less complicated approaches to AIDS therapy.

## C. INTERNALIZATION OF HUMAN ANTIBODIES AGAINST HIV-1

To determine whether HIV-1-infected T lymphocytes are able to internalize HIV-neutralizing human antibodies, antibodies to *env* 2–3[26,25] were $^{125}$I-labeled and incubated with noninfected or HIV-1-infected T lymphocytes (Table 3). Antibodies to *env* 2–3 were obtained from human sera which showed strong HIV-1-neutralizing activity, by purification on a yeast recombinant gp120-Sepharose 4B column.[26,25] The recombinant gp120 (protein *env* 2–3) used in the procedure of purification was produced in yeast and is not glycosylated; therefore, antibody *env* 2–3 does not recognize the conformational epitopes of gp120. A fraction of antibodies was internalized by T lymphocytes on the third day after HIV infection (syncytia formation), but not on the first day of infection.[43] Eighty percent of the internalized antibody was found in the cell nucleus (4250 molecules/cell nucleus). Noninfected T lymphocytes did not internalize the antibody. $^{125}$I-labeled IgG-fraction from con-

## TABLE 3
## Internalization of Human Neutralizing
## Antibodies Labeled with [125]I after
## 24-h Incubation with Noninfected or
## HIV-1-Infected T Lymphocytes

| Day after infection[c] | Molecules per cell[a] SupT1[b] | |
| | Cytoplasm | Nucleus |
| --- | --- | --- |
| **Antibodies to *env* 2-3** | | |
| Noninfected | 250 | 30 |
| 1 | 260 ± 25 | 400 ± 40 |
| 3 | 800 ± 200 | 4,500 ± 1,000 |
| **Human IgG from HIV-negative patients** | | |
| Noninfected | 230 | 40 |
| 1 | 220 | 30 |
| 3 | 220 | 40 |

[a] Mean + SD from three experiments.
[b] T lymphocytes-SupT1 infected with HIV-1 (HXB-2).
[c] Day after infection is the day when the [125]I-mAb was added to the medium.

trol sera of HIV-1-negative people was not internalized. The results indicate that a fraction of antibodies synthesized during natural human infection is able to penetrate the HIV-1-infected cell. The possibility that nonspecific adsorption of human IgG to cellular structures occurs during fractionation is eliminated, since [125]I-IgG isolated from HIV-1-negative patients did not enter infected T lymphocytes (Table 3).

Whether antibodies to *env* 2–3 are internalized "using" the same epitopes as mAb 5023 is yet unknown. The fact that the core antigen RAF and the preceding residue G are present in SF$_2$ gp120 which was used to purify antibodies to *env* 2–3 supports such a possibility. In fact, the sequence GRAF represents a C terminal part of the sequence GPGRAF which is frequently present in the principal neutralizing determinant of gp120 expressed by different isolates which was found to induce antibodies neutralizing divergent isolates.[28,29]

Since [125]I-labeled mAb targeting to the nucleus of cancer cells were found to destroy DNA effectively, we can suggest that chromatin of HIV-1-infected cells may represent a new target for radiotherapy of HIV-infected patients. Theoretically, therapy of HIV patients with mAb targeting to the nucleus should be less toxic than analogous therapy of cancer patients. The reason for such a prediction is that cancer antigens are also expressed in lower amounts on normal cells. In contrast, the gp120 used as the target antigen for radiotherapy of AIDS would be expressed only on

HIV-infected cells and on the virus. Using effectively internalized and radioactively labeled mAb, like mAb 5023, we should be able to destroy the population of infected cells.

Pincus et al.[33] constructed immunotoxins using serum-derived anti-HIV gp160 antibodies and showed that these complexes were able to kill HIV-infected cells. Finding human antibodies able to penetrate HIV-1-infected lymphocytes stresses the potential importance of such antibodies in protection against AIDS development. We suggest that antibodies able to penetrate HIV-infected cells may represent a quantitatively variable fraction of antibodies synthesized during natural human infection. It may be speculated that internalized antibodies may block synthesis of gp120 inside the infected cells and thereby inhibit syncytia formation as well as reassembly of the virus. If such a mechanism takes place *in vivo,* it is possible that HIV-infected patients able to produce the internalizable antibodies may have a better chance to survive than those who synthesize antibodies unable to penetrate the cell. If the last hypothesis is confirmed, gp120 epitope(s) that mediate internalization of antibodies may represent the key for developing effective vaccines. Since internalized antibodies are localized in cytoplasm as well as in the nucleus, we can suggest that mAb conjugated with a transcriptional/replicational inhibitor-ligand or a radioactive ligand may be used in different therapeutic approaches.

## III. IMMUNOLOGICAL CROSS-REACTIVITY OF ANTI-HIV-1-gp120 INTERNALIZABLE ANTIBODIES WITH BREAST CARCINOMA ANTIGENS

The specificities of HIV-neutralizing (Section II) mAb and human antibodies internalized by HIV-1-infected T lymphocytes were tested by using several tumor cell lines, supposedly negative controls since they do not express gp120 antigen. Unexpectedly, mAb 5023 against envelope protein gp120 of HIV-1, which is internalized by HIV-infected cells, was also found to penetrate breast carcinoma cells, but not melanoma or colorectal carcinoma cells.[51] The experiments resulted in identification of breast carcinoma antigens which show immunological crossreactivity with HIV-1 antigens.[47]

### A. IMMUNOFLUORESCENCE DETECTION OF mAb 5023 AGAINST THE HIV-1 gp120 INSIDE THE BREAST CARCINOMA CELLS

Breast carcinoma SKBr 5, MCF7, melanoma A875, and colorectal carcinoma SW1116 cells were incubated with mAb developed against the overlapping regions of the neutralizing V3 loop of HIV-1 envelope protein gp120 (see Section II) followed by incubation with fluoresceine-labeled sheep anti-mouse IgG (Figure 1).[47] mAb 5023 against gp120 region 308 to 322 was the only mAb which was internalized by breast carcinoma cells.

Internalization of mAb 5023 by breast carcinoma cells was tested by indirect immunofluorescence staining of cells infected with HIV-1. After 15 min of SKBr 5 cell incubation with mAb 5023 at 0°C, an immunofluorescence ring surrounded

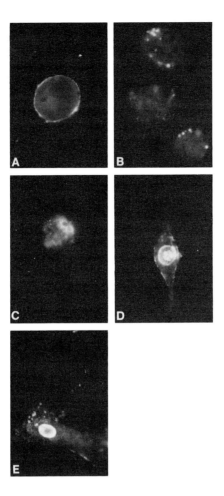

**FIGURE 1.** Immunofluorescence staining of SKBr 5 (A to D) and MCF7 (E) breast carcinoma cells with fluoresceine-conjugated sheep anti-mouse IgG after incubation with mAb 5023 at 0°C for 15 min (A), or at 37°C for 1 h (B), 3 h (C), and 24 h (D, E).

breast carcinoma cells, indicating that mAb 5023 bound to a cell surface-associated molecule (Figure 1A). After 15 min to 1 h of incubation at 37°C, fluorescent spots were detected inside the cytoplasm (Figure 1B), which suggests that the mAb was internalized and localized in the endosomal vesicles. After longer exposure (3 to 5 h), the fluorescence of cytoplasm became more diffuse and seemed to be distributed within the cytoplasm and the nucleus (Figure 1C). After 24 h of incubation of breast carcinoma cells, the strong fluorescence of the nucleus was easily distinguishable from the much weaker fluorescence of the cytoplasm (Figure 1D). The predominantly nuclear location of mAb 5023 was also observed in MCF7 cells (Figure 1E). mAb 5023, after 24 h of incubation, was undetectable in control colorectal carci-

**TABLE 4**
**Internalization of $^{125}$I-mAb 5023**
**Against gp120 and of Human**
**Neutralizing Antibodies after 24-h**
**Incubation with Breast Carcinoma**
**Cell Line SKBr 5**

|  | Molecules per cell[a] | |
|---|---|---|
| $^{125}$I-mAb or antibody | Cytoplasm | Nucleus[b] |
| 5023 | 1,890 | 5,450 |
| 5025 | 350 | 200 |
| VM77 | 60 | 20 |
| 0.5β | 35 | 60 |
| Antibodies to *env* 2-3 | 2,456 | 10,080 |
| Human IgG | 50 | 45 |
| (HIV-1-negative) | | |

[a]   Mean from four experiments; SD = 10% for
      mAb, 15% for antibody *env* 2-3.
[b]   Molecules bound to the chromatin, nucleo-
      plasm, and nuclear membranes. Chromatin bound
      85 to 95% of the nuclear $^{125}$I-mAb 5023.

noma cells (not shown). mAb 5025, 0.5β, and VM77 were undetectable in breast
carcinoma cells (not shown). The results indicated that only one mAb, mAb 5023,
was internalized by SKBr 5 cells, which eliminates a possibility of nonspecific
penetration of breast carcinoma cells by the anti-HIV-1 antibody.[47]

## B.  INTRACELLULAR LOCALIZATION OF $^{125}$I-mAb 5023 BY BREAST CARCINOMA CELLS

Intracellular uptake of mAb 5023 by breast carcinoma cells was confirmed by
fractionation of cells exposed to $^{125}$I-labeled mAb (Table 4).[47] $^{125}$I-mAb 5023 was
internalized by the cells and localized in the cytoplasm and in the nucleus (Table
4). None of the other mAb tested against gp120 were internalized by breast carcinoma cells.

Electrophoretic analysis of the internalized $^{125}$I-mAb 5023 indicated that, after
24 h of incubation, $^{125}$I-mAb 5023 extracted from the cytoplasm and from the
chromatin exhibited the same molecular weight of both heavy and light chains as
did the native mAb (Figure 2). Thus mAb 5023 penetrated breast carcinoma cell
nuclei in a nondegraded form.[47]

## C.  IDENTIFICATION OF BREAST CARCINOMA ANTIGENS WHICH CROSS-REACT WITH THE INTERNALIZING mAb AGAINST gp120

To determine whether internalization of mAb 5023 is mediated by a specific
antigen, mAb 5023 and four other mAb were tested in Western blotting for reactivity
with plasma membrane proteins and chromatin proteins of breast carcinoma SKBr 5

$^{125}$I-MAb5023/SkBr5

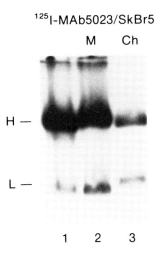

FIGURE 2. Autoradiographic detection of free $^{125}$I-mAb 5023 (lane 1) and $^{125}$I-mAb 5023 accumulated in the cytoplasm (lane 2) and in the chromatin (lane 3) after 24 h incubation with SKBr 5 cells. Cytoplasm and chromatin were prepared from $5 \times 10^6$ cells.

cells (Figure 2).[47] When the electrophoresis of proteins was performed in 7.5% polyacrylamide gel, the mAb 5023 reacted with a major 160,000 $M_r$ (p160) antigen of plasma membranes, a minor band of the $M_r$ 80,000 (p80), and a sharp band of the $M_r$ 45,000 (p45) (Figure 3A; lane 2). Other mAb against gp120 recognized only p45, but not p160 and p80 (Figure 3A; lanes 3 to 5). None of the protein bands detected in a plasma membrane fraction were detected in the chromatin (Figure 3A; lane 1).

In a 13% polyacrylamide gel, a major protein-band of the $M_r$ 24,000 (p24) was detected in both the cell membrane fraction and in the chromatin by mAb 5023 (Figure 3B; lanes 3 and 4). Other mAb tested did not recognize the p24 (Figure 3B; lanes 1, 2, and 5 to 8).

Antigens p160, p80, and p45 in the membrane fraction (Figure 4A) and p24 in both the membrane and the chromatin fractions were also detected in the other breast carcinoma cell lines (SKBr 3, MCF7, BT20, and CAMA) (Figure 4B). In the chromatin, in addition to the 24,000 $M_r$ protein, a 23,000 $M_r$ minor band was detected. Neither mAb 5023 (Figure 4) nor any other mAb (not shown) recognized any of the plasma membrane antigens in colorectal carcinoma SW1116 (Figure 4A; lane 8), lung carcinoma SW900 (Figure 4A; lane 6), or melanoma 451 Lu (Figure 4A; lane 7). In melanoma cell line 451 Lu, but not in the other cell lines tested, a low expression of p24/p23 was detected in the chromatin (Figure 4B; lane 5).[47]

It is likely that p160 may represent a dimeric form of p80. We also cannot eliminate the possibility that p45 and p24 in the cell membrane represent degradation products of p160. Alternatively, all of the proteins recognized by mAb 5023 may originate from a one precursor protein. The relative amount of p160, p80, and p24

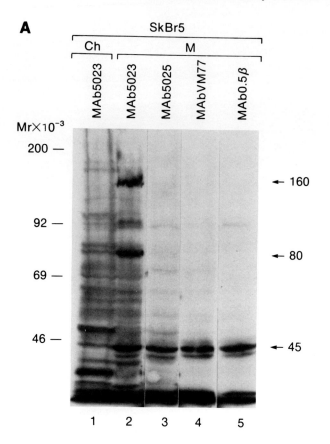

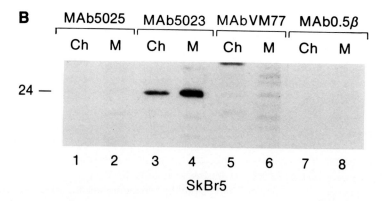

**FIGURE 3.** Western blotting of different mAb against V3 loop of HIV-1 gp120 with membrane (M) and chromatin (Ch) proteins of SKBr 5 cells separated in a 7.5% (A) or 13% (B) polyacrylamide gel.

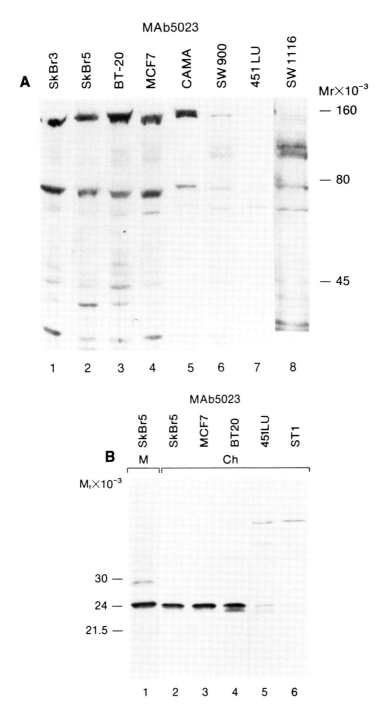

**FIGURE 4.** Western blotting of mAb 5023 with membrane (M) and chromatin (Ch) proteins of different cell lines separated in 7.5% (A) or 13% (B) polyacrylamide gel.

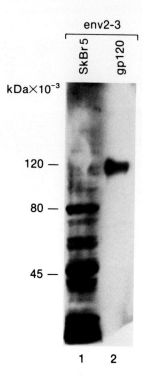

**FIGURE 5.**   Western blotting of human HIV-1-neutralizing antibodies to *env* 2-3 with SKBr 5 breast carcinoma membrane proteins (lane 1) and HIV-1 gp120 (lane 2). Proteins are separated in 7.5% polyacrylamide gel.

was similar in samples obtained from independent experiments, while the relative amount of p45 varied from experiment to experiment.

Immunoprecipitation of SKBr 5 breast carcinoma cell plasma membrane with mAb 5023 revealed proteins p160, p45 (Figure 5), and p24 (not shown). Protein p80 observed in Western blotting was not immunoprecipitated, which suggests that monomer p80 in native form may not be recognized by mAb 5023. Since mAb 5023 was the only mAb which was able to enter breast carcinoma cells and translocate to the nucleus and, simultaneously, the only mAb able to recognize p160 (and p80), it is likely that p160 (and p80) expresses a specific epitope which is critical for mAb internalization. A nonspecific adsorption of the cell membrane-bound [125]I-mAb 5023 to the chromatin during cell fractionation may be eliminated, since p160, p80, and p45 represent the specific markers of the cell membrane fraction and are not found in the chromatin.

The chromatin did not show any trace of p160, p80, and p45 which eliminates the possibility that the cytoplasmic protein p24 attached nonspecifically to the chromatin during cell fractionation. We suspect that chromatin-bound p24 may bind the mAb 5023 translocated to the nucleus.[47]

## D. BREAST CARCINOMA CELL ANTIGEN CROSS-REACTIVITY AND INTERNALIZATION OF HUMAN HIV-1 NEUTRALIZING SERA

Since mAb 5023 was developed against a synthetic peptide,[24,25] it seemed likely that an artificial conformation of this peptide might induce an antibody of the idiotype very different from that induced by the same peptide localized inside the native structure of *env* gp120 of HIV-1. Alternatively, if the conformational structure of the peptide used to induce mAb 5023 was not different from that present in the hypervariable loop of gp120, then antibodies of the idiotypic homology to mAb 5023 would be expressed in HIV-infected patients.

To determine whether antibodies crossreactive with breast carcinoma antigens are also produced by AIDS patients, we have tested human antibodies to gp120. Human sera which showed strong HIV-1-neutralizing activity were collected and purified on a yeast recombinant gp120-Sepharose 4B column, yielding the human antibody to *env* 2-3.[26,27] The recombinant gp120 (protein *env* 2-3) used in the procedure of purification was produced in yeast and is not glycosylated, and therefore, antibody *env* 2-3 does not recognize the conformational epitopes of gp120.

HIV-1 neutralizing human antibodies to *env* 2-3[28] reacted in Western blotting with 80,000 $M_r$ and 45,000 $M_r$ breast carcinoma cell membrane antigens[47] (Figure 5). A fraction of [125]I-labeled antibodies to *env* 2-3 was internalized by breast carcinoma cells and localized in the cytoplasm and in the nucleus (Table 4). Thus, internalizable antibodies are produced in natural human HIV infection. Since the human antibodies also recognize breast carcinoma antigens p80 and p45, it is likely that epitopes expressed by those proteins are critical for internalization.

## E. UPTAKE OF mAb 5023 BY ISOLATED NUCLEI

[125]I-mAb 5023, when incubated with nuclei isolated from SKBr 5 breast carcinoma cells, was found to enter the nucleus and bind to the chromatin (Table 5).[47] In control experiments, [125]I-BSA was used instead of [125]I-mAb. The [125]I-BSA did not enter the nucleus. BSA ($M_r$ 65,000) is a much smaller molecule than immunoglobulin ($M_r$ 155,000), and, therefore, a passive diffusion of mAb due to nuclei damage during preparation — or a nonspecific adsorption of immunoglobulins to the chromatin during nucleus fractionation — may be eliminated. To determine whether mAb 5023 is taken up by the nucleus through the mediation of the *N*-acetylglucosamine-bound nuclear membrane receptor, which was found to mediate nuclear translocation of SV40 large T antigen and other proteins which contain the nuclear localization signal, the effect of WGA on nuclear uptake of mAb 5023 was tested. Nuclear translocation of mAb 5023 was significantly blocked by WGA (Table 5), suggesting that the nuclear membrane receptor may be involved in intranuclear translocation of this mAb.

## F. CONCLUSIONS

Cross-reactivity of mAb 5023 and human antibodies against HIV-1 gp120 with breast carcinoma antigens represents a phenomenon which can be explained either by a conformational or structural homology of HIV envelope protein and breast

**TABLE 5**
**Effect of Wheat Germ Agglutinin (WGA) on Nuclear
Uptake of $^{125}$I-mAb 5023 in a Cell-Free System[a]**

| WGA concentration (mg/ml) | Nuclear membranes | $^{125}$I-mAb 5023 incorporation[b] (cpm) | |
|---|---|---|---|
| | | Nucleoplasm | Chromatin |
| 0 | 11,700 | 1,530 | 100,000 |
| 0.625 | 10,440 | 950 | 87,000 |
| 1.25 | 9,950 | 860 | 75,800 |
| 2.5 | 5,840 | 610 | 42,900 |

[a]  Five $\times$ $10^6$ nuclei/ml were incubated for 1 h at room temperature with $^{125}$I-mAb.

[b]  Mean from three experiments; SD = 5 to 8%.

carcinoma antigens. Recently Khalife et al.[48] reported an immunological cross-reactivity between the HIV-1 virion infectivity factor (vif) and a 170 $M_r$ surface antigen of *S. mansoni*. However, there is no antigenic cross-reactivity between HIV-1 structural proteins and *S. mansoni* antigens. Antibodies to HIV were also found to be associated with malaria.[49,50] Breast carcinoma antigen p160 (and its monomeric form p80) deserves special attention, since it seems to contain an epitope whose recognition is critical for mAb internalization. Since the internalized mAb 5023 was developed against a short region of HIV-1 gp120 covering amino acids 308 to 322, it is likely that this region, particularly the sequence GRAF which represents the epitope recognized by mAb 5023 must also be expressed in breast carcinoma p160. Alternatively, gp160 may express a conformation epitope homologous to that of HIV-1 gp120. It is noteworthy that the $M_r$ 160,000 of breast carcinoma antigen correlates to the $M_r$ of the HIV-1 precursor of gp120. Whether the proteins of breast carcinoma that cross-react with mAb against HIV-1 gp120 represent products of human or retrovirus genes is currently unknown. We suspect that a retrovirus of strong homology to HIV-1 may be present in breast carcinomas. Internalization of $^{125}$I antibodies to *env* 2-3, which represent a fraction of the human HIV-1 neutralizing antibodies able to recognize the unglycosylated form of gp120,[27] by breast carcinoma cells as well[46] as by HIV-1-infected T cells,[43] suggests that internalizable antibodies represent a fraction of antibodies synthesized by AIDS patients. We suggest that antibodies able to penetrate HIV-infected cells may play a critical role in inhibition of syncytia formation and in the process of virus neutralization (see Section II).

# REFERENCES

1. **Barré-Sinoussi, F., Chermann, J. C., Rey, F., et al.,** Isolation of a T-lymphotrophic retrovirus from a patient at risk for AIDS, *Science,* 220, 868, 1983.
2. **Popovic, M., Sarngadharan, M. G., Read, E., and Gallo, R. C.,** Detection, isolation, and continuous production of cytopathic retroviruses (HTLV III) from patients with AIDS and pre-AIDS, *Science,* 224, 497, 1984.
3. **Gallo, R. C., Salahuddin, S. Z., Popovic, M., et al.,** Frequent detection and isolation of cytopathic retroviruses (HTLV-III) from patients with AIDS or at risk for AIDS, *Science,* 224, 500, 1984.
4. **Clavel, F., Guetard, D., Brun-Vezinet, F., et al.,** Isolation of a new human retrovirus from West African patients with AIDS, *Science,* 233, 343, 1986.
5. **Özel, M., Pauli, G., and Gelderblom, H. R.,** The organization of the envelope projections on the surface of HIV, *Arch. Virol.,* 100, 255, 1988.
6. **Gelderblom, H. R., Hausmann, E. H. S., Özel, M., Pauli, G., and Koch, M. A.,** Fine structure of LAV/HTLV III and immunolocalization of structural proteins, *Virology,* 156, 171, 1987.
7. **Grewe, C., Beck, A., and Gelderblom, H. R.,** HIV: early virus-cell interactions, *J. AIDS,* 3, 965, 1990.
8. **Klatzmann, D., Champagne, E., Chamaret, S., et al.,** T lymphocyte T4 molecule behaves as the receptor for human retrovirus LAV, *Nature,* 312, 767, 1984.
9. **Lasky, L. A., Nakamura, G., Smith, D. H., Fennic, C., Shimasaki, C., Patzer, E., Berman, P., Gregory, T., and Capon, D. J.,** Delineation of a region of the human immunodeficiency virus type 1 gp120 glycoprotein critical for interaction with the CD4 receptor, *Cell,* 50, 975, 1987.
10. **Maddon, P. J., Dalgleish, A. G., McDougal, J. S., Clapham, P. R., Weiss, R. A., and Axel, R.,** The T4 gene encodes the AIDS virus receptor and is expressed in the immune system and the brain, *Cell,* 47, 333, 1986.
11. **McDougal, J. S., Nicholson, J. K. A., Cross, G. D., Cort, S. P., Kennedy, M. S., and Mawle, A. C.,** Binding of the human retrovirus HTLV-II/LAV/ARV/HIV to the CD4 (T4) molecule: conformation dependence, epitope mapping, antibody inhibition, and potential for idiotypic mimicry, *J. Immunol.,* 137, 2937, 1986.
12. **Sattentau, Q. J. and Weiss, R. A.,** The CD4 antigen: physiological ligand and HIV receptor, *Cell,* 52, 631, 1988.
13. **Marsh, M. and Dalgleish, A.,** How do human immunodeficiency viruses enter cells?, *Immunol. Today,* 8, 369, 1987.
14. **Sinangil, F., Loyter, A., and Volsky, D. J.,** Quantitative measurement of fusion between human immunodeficiency virus and cultured cells using membrane fusion dequenching, *F.E.B.S. Lett.,* 239, 88, 1988.
15. **Ribas, T., Hase, E., Hunter, D., Fritz, D., Khan, N., and Burke, D.,** HIV Enters Cells by Fusion with Cell Membrane, paper presented at the IVth International Conference on AIDS, Stockholm, 1988, 1025.
16. **Kulkosky, J. and Skalka, A. M.,** HIV DNA integration: observations and inferences, *J. Acquired Immune Deficiency Syndromes,* 3, 839, 1990.
17. **Litson, J., Feinberg, M., and Reyes, G.,** Induction of CD-4-dependent cell fusion by the HTLV III/LAV envelope antigen, *Nature,* 323, 725, 1986.
18. **Matthews, T. F., Langlois, A. J., Robey, W. G., Chang, N. T., Gallo, R. C., Fischinger, P. J., and Bolognesi, D. P.,** Restricted neutralization of divergent human T-lymphotropic virus type III isolate by antibodies to the major envelope glycoprotein, *Proc. Natl. Acad. Sci. U.S.A.,* 83, 9709, 1986.
19. **Kenealy, W. R., Matthews, T. J., Ganfield, M. -C., Langlois, A. J., Waselefsky, D. M., and Petteway, S. R.,** Antibodies from human immunodeficiency virus-infected individuals bind to a short amino acid sequence that elicits neutralizing antibodies in animals, *AIDS Res. Human Retroviruses,* 5, 173, 1989.

20. **Goudsmit, J., Debouck, C., Meloen, R. H., Smit, L., Bakker, M., Asher, D. M., Wolff, A. V., Gibbs, C. J., Jr., and Gajdusek, D. C.,** Human immunodeficiency virus type 1 neutralization epitope with conserved architecture elicits early type-specific antibodies in experimentally infected chimpanzees, *Proc. Natl. Acad. Sci. U.S.A.,* 85, 4478, 1988.

21. **Cheng-Mayer, C., Homsy, J., Evans, L. A., and Levy, J. A.,** Identification of human immunodeficiency virus subtypes with distinct patterns of sensitivity to serum neutralization, *Proc. Natl. Acad. Sci. U.S.A.,* 85, 2815, 1988.

22. **Ho, D. D., Sarngagharan, M. G., Hirsch, M. S., Schooley, R. T., Rota, T. R., Kennedy, R. C., Chanh, T. C., and Sato, V. L.,** Human immunodeficiency virus neutralizing antibodies recognize several conserved domains of the envelope glycoproteins, *J. Virol.,* 61, 2024, 1987.

23. **Langedijk, J. P. M., Back, N. K. T., Durda, P. J., Goudsmit, J., and Meleon, R. H.,** Neutralizing activity of anti-peptide antibodies against the principal neutralization domain of human immunodeficiency virus type 1, *J. Gen. Virol.,* 72, 2519, 1991.

24. **Durda, P. J., Bacheler, L., Clapham, P., Jenoski, A. M., Leece, B., Matthews, T. J., McKnight, A., Pomerantz, R., Rayner, M., and Weinhold, K. J.,** HIV-1 neutralizing monoclonal antibodies induced by a synthetic peptide, *AIDS Res. Human Retroviruses,* 6, 1115, 1990.

25. **Langedijk, J. P. M., Back, N. K. T., Durda, P. J., Goudsmit, J., and Meloen, R. H.,** Neutralizing activity of anti-peptide antibodies against the principal neutralization domain of human immunodeficiency virus type 1, *J. Gen. Virol.,* 72, 2519, 1991.

26. **Haigwood, N. L., Barker, C. B., Higgins, K. W., Skiles, P. V., Moore, G. K., Mann, K. A., Lee, D. R., Eichberg, J. W., and Steimer, K. S.,** Evidence for neutralizing antibodies directed against conformational epitopes of HIV-1 gp120, *Vaccines,* Cold Spring Harbor Laboratory Press, New York, 1990.

27. **Steimer, K. S., Scandella, C. J., Skiles, P. V., Haigwood, N. L.,** Neutralization of divergent HIV-1 isolates by conformation-dependent human antibodies to gp120, *Science,* 254, 105, 1991.

28. **Javaherian, V., Langlois, A. J., LaRosa, G. J., Profy, A. T., Bolognesi, D. P., Hertihy, W. C., Putney, S., and Matthews, T.,** Broadly neutralizing antibodies elicited by the hypervariable neutralizing determinant of HIV-1, *Science,* 250, 1590, 1990.

29. **Ohno, T., Terada, M., Yoneda, Y., Shea, K., Chambers, R. F., Stroka, D. M., Nakamura, M., and Kufe, D. W.,** A broadly neutralizing monoclonal antibody that recognizes the V3 region of human immunodeficiency virus type 1 glycoprotein gp120, *Proc. Natl. Acad. Sci. U.S.A.,* 88, 10726, 1991.

30. **Chaudhary, V. K., Mizukami, T., Fuerst, T. R., FitzGerald, D. J., Moss, B., Pastan, I., and Berger, E. A.,** Selective killing of HIV-infected cells by recombinant human CD4-*Pseudomonas* exotoxin hybrid protein, *Nature,* 335, 369, 1988.

31. **Till, M. A., Ghetie, V., Gregory, T., Patzer, E. J., Porter, J. P., Uhr, J. W., Capon, D. J., and Vitetta, E. S.,** HIV-infected cells are killed by rCD4-ricin A chain, *Science,* 242, 1166, 1988.

32. **Pincus, S. M., Wherly, K., and Cherebzo, B.,** Treatment of HIV tissue culture infection with monoclonal antibody-ricin A chain conjugates, *J. Immunol.,* 142, 3070, 1989.

33. **Pincus, S. M., Cole, R. L., Marsh, E. M., Lake, D., Masuko, Y., Durda, P. J., and McClure, J.,** In vitro efficacy of anti-HIV immunotoxins targeted by various antibodies to the envelope protein, *J. Immunol.,* 146, 4215, 1991.

34. **Matsushita, S., Koito, A., Maeda, Y., Mattoni, T., and Takatsuki, K.,** Selective killing of HIV-infected cells by anti-gp120 immunotoxins, *AIDS Res. Human Retroviruses,* 6, 193, 1990.

35. **Till, M. A., Zolla-Pazner, S., Gorny, M. K., Patton, J. S., Uhr, J. W., and Vitetta, E. S.,** Human immunodeficiency virus-infected T cells and monocytes are killed by monoclonal human anti-gp41 antibodies coupled to ricin A chain, *Proc. Natl. Acad. Sci. U.S.A.,* 86, 1987, 1989.

36. **Endo, Y., Mitsui, K., Matizuki, M., and Tsurugi, K.,** The mechanisms of action of ricin and related toxic lectins on eukaryotic ribosomes, *J. Biol. Chem.,* 202, 5908, 1987.

37. **Endo, Y. and Tsurugi, K.,** RNA N-glycosidase activity of ricin A chain. Mechanism of action of the toxic lectin ricin on eukaryotic ribosomes, *J. Biol. Chem.,* 262, 8128, 1987.

38. **Vitetta, E. S., Krolick, K. A., Miyama-Inaba, M., Cushley, W., and Uhr, J. W.,** Immunotoxins: a new approach to cancer therapy, *Science,* 219, 644, 1083.

39. **Blakey, D. C. and Thorpe, P. E.,** An overview of therapy with immunotoxins containing ricin or its A chain, *Antibody Immunoconj. Radiopharm.,* 1, 1, 1988.

40. **Rakowicz-Szulczynska, E., Otwiaski, D., Rodeck, U., and Koprowski, H.,** Epidermal growth factor (EGF) and monoclonal antibody to cell surface EGF receptor bind to the same chromatin receptor, *Arch. Biochem. Biophys.,* 268, 456, 1989.

41. **Rakowicz-Szulczynska, E. and Koprowski, H.,** Nuclear uptake of monoclonal antibody to a surface glycoprotein and its effect on transcription, *Arch. Biochem. Biophys.,* 271, 366, 1989.

42. **Rakowicz-Szulczynska, E., Steplewski, Z., and Koprowski, H.,** Nuclear translocation of monoclonal antibody directed against cell surface carbohydrate Y determinant, *Am. J. Pathol.,* 141, 938–947, 1992.

43. **Rakowicz-Szulczynska, E., Raso, V., Kacsmarski, W., and Durda, P. J.,** unpublished data.

44. **Skinner, M. A., Ting, R., Langlois, A. J., Weinhold, K. J., Lyerly, H. K., Javaherian, K., and Matthews, T. J.,** Characteristics of a neutralizing monoclonal antibody to the HIV envelope glycoprotein, *AIDS Res. Human Retroviruses,* 4, 187, 1988.

45. **Harrison, G. S., Long, C. J., Maxwell, F., Glode, M., and Maxwell, I. M.,** Inhibition of HIV production in cells containing an integrated HIV-regulated diphtheria toxin A chain gene, *AIDS Res. Human Retroviruses,* 8, 39, 1992.

46. **Baltimore, D.,** Intracellular immunization, *Nature,* 335, 7395, 1988.

47. **Rakowicz-Szulczynska, E., Durda, P. J., and Kaczmarski, W.,** Immunological cross-reactivity between HIV-1 gp120 and breast carcinoma cell surface and chromatin antigens, submitted.

48. **Khalife, J., Grzych, J. M., Pierce, R., Ameisen, J. C., Schacht, A. M., Gras-Masse, H., Tartar, A., Lecocq, J. P., and Capron, A.,** Immunological cross-reactivity between the human immunodeficiency virus type 1 virion infectivity factor and a 170 kDa surface antigen of *Schistoma mansoni, J. Exp. Med.,* 172, 1001, 1990.

49. **Biggar, R. J., Johnson, B. K., Oster, C., Sarin, P. S., Ocheng, D., Tukei, P., Nsanze, H., Alexander, S., Bonder, A. J., Siongok, T. A., Gallo, R. C., and Blattner, W. A.,** Regional variation in prevalence of antibody against human T-lymphotropic virus types I and II in Kenya East Africa, *Int. J. Cancer,* 35, 763, 1985.

50. **Biggar, R. J., Melbye, M., Sarin, P. S., Demedts, P., Deacollette, C., Gigase, P. L., Kestens, L., Bodner, A. J., Leopold Palulu, W. J. S., and Blattner, W. A.,** ELISA HTLV retroviruses antibody reactivity associated with malaria and immune complexes in healthy Africans, *Lancet,* ii, 520, 1985.

*Index*

# INDEX

## A

## B

# C